HOW TO LEARN AND TEACH
IN MEDICAL SCHOOL:
A LEARNER–CENTERED APPROACH

HOW TO LEARN AND TEACH IN MEDICAL SCHOOL:
A Learner-Centered Approach

By

MARK E. QUIRK, ED.D.

Professor of Family and Community Medicine
Assistant Dean for Student Academic Achievement
University of Massachusetts Medical School
Worcester, Massachusetts

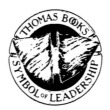

CHARLES C THOMAS • PUBLISHER
Springfield • Illinois • U.S.A.

Published and Distributed Throughout the World by

CHARLES C THOMAS • PUBLISHER
2600 South First Street
Springfield, Illinois 62794-9265

© *1994 by* CHARLES C THOMAS • PUBLISHER
ISBN 0-398-05925-X (cloth)
ISBN 0-398-06512-8 (paper)
Library of Congress Catalog Card Number: 94-21620

With THOMAS BOOKS *careful attention is given to all details of manufact
and design. It is the Publisher's desire to present books that are satisfactory as to
physical qualities and artistic possibilities and appropriate for their particula*
THOMAS BOOKS *will be true to those laws of quality that assure a good
and good will.*

Printed in the United States of America
SC-R-3

Library of Congress Cataloging-in-Publication Data

Quirk, Mark E.
    How to learn and teach in medical school : a learner-centered
approach / by Mark E. Quirk.
        p.   cm.
    Includes bibliographical references and index.
    ISBN 0-398-05925-X. — 0-398-06512-8 (pbk.)
    1. Medical education. I. Title.
R735.Q57   1994
610'.71'1 — dc20   94-21620
                                                                              CIP

For Jan, Mike, Shaun, and Kev

PREFACE

This book can be used by students, faculty, and administrators to enhance the process of medical education. Medical students can use it to develop and refine their learning skills, assess their individual learning needs, identify resources to meet these needs, and to prepare themselves for critical learning events and transitions. Faculty can use this book to understand the learning process and develop teaching skills, thereby providing a framework for critically assessing how they teach. Administrators can use it to expose inadequacies in the medical education process and to strengthen the teaching and learning environment.

Certain chapters of this book could serve as required readings for a medical school course on learning. The development and implementation of such a course, and the commensurate application of the espoused principles of learning and teaching to the educational process, would signal true medical educational reform. It would signify that critical attention is being paid to those aspects of learning medicine thought to be crucial: reading the literature, self-directedness, critical thinking/problem solving, lifelong learning and creativity. Such a course would be as important as any basic science course or clinical rotation to the training of future physicians who would use these skills throughout their professional lives.

The book also could serve as a foundation for faculty development with medical educators. In this regard, Part I provides insight into *how* medical students learn and has significant implications for teaching. Parts II and III provide *practical guidelines* for teaching and curriculum development from a learner-centered perspective.

M.E.Q.

INTRODUCTION

Learner-centered medical education focuses attention on the student. This title implies a rather radical shift from the status quo which focuses primarily on medical content.

Several problems with a *content-oriented* approach have developed. First, much of the knowledge gained in medical school will be invalid, or at the very least outdated, by the time the student enters practice. Alfred North Whitehead, an eminent educator in the early twentieth century, reminds us of the ephemeral nature of knowledge when he states: "Knowledge does not keep any better than fish" (1929, p. 98). This rather unappetizing notion is particularly applicable to medicine, where the half-life of knowledge is more short-lived than in most disciplines. Concerning the medical literature, which is a repository for this knowledge, John S. Billings, the founder of *Index Medicus* states: "Nine-tenths at least, of it, becomes worthless and of no interest, within ten years after the date of its publication, and much of it is so when it first appears" (1887, p. 63).

A second, related problem with the content approach to medical education is that because the volume of information continues to escalate at such a rapid pace, there is *too much* content to be learned. This problem has been raised by many medical educators. As Derek Bok says: "The growth of scientific knowledge itself is pressing hard against the familiar notion of what it means to think like a doctor. The constant flow of new discoveries makes impossible demands on human memory" (1984, p. 36). Although many have alluded to the problem, few have offered viable solutions.

A third problem with this current orientation is that the heavy volume of content to be learned (along with the accompanying educational methods chosen to *bestow* it) has completely *turned off* many students. Learners enter with high expectations for learning and teaching and shortly lose them along with their motivation to learn. The ever-increasing volume of information presented forces students to superficially learn material which they view as only peripherally related to their impending professional lives. The *system* also forces them to neglect learning some of the content which they may feel is relevant to the practice of medicine because it *won't appear on an exam.*

Finally, a content-oriented approach fails to prepare learners to continue to learn on their own. With such an emphasis on content, the *process* of learning is neglected and often devalued. Despite the medical information implosion, and *lip service* paid to *self-directed, lifelong learning,* such a prerequisite to competent clinical practice is not adequately addressed.

Learner-centered medical education is a viable alternative which addresses the shortcomings of a content-based curriculum. It is not simply a shifting or re-packaging of content (e.g., organ-based approach) which is commonplace today in curricular reform. Instead, it focuses on preparing the student (and ultimately the physician) to be a competent, effective, efficient, and motivated learner. The emphasis is on the development of a set of learning skills which will enable the medical student to learn in medical school *and beyond* from teachers, from him/herself and from patients.

Because learning content is secondary to learning skills, the inevitable demise of *truth* is no longer a problem. It is fully expected that this will occur and the learner is poised for this occurrence. With the pressure off the teacher to convey, and the student to learn *all* of the content, both can be selective in the content chosen as the raw material for developing necessary learning skills. With the emphasis on learning skills and the reduction of volume, true learning with understanding can take place.

The experience of greater and deeper mastery along with exposure to teaching methods which are engaging and exciting will restore motivation and creativity to the medical students's learning experience. For this type of learning to take place, teaching must take on a new meaning. Teachers must not only know how to plan a learning experience but must prepare the student to plan a learning experience for her/himself. Teachers must become *flexible* in the use of teaching behaviors depending upon the needs of the learner.

Finally, for learner-centered medical education to flourish it must be set in a *proper milieu.* This entails a setting where the learner and learning come first, growth on all levels is fostered, and differences among learners respected.

Learner-centered medical education is the inevitable next step in the process of revitalizing medical education. In this book some principles and guidelines for undertaking such revitalization are put forth. It will be up to faculty, administrators, and the students themselves to apply these principles and guidelines to the learning-teaching process.

ACKNOWLEDGMENTS

I wish to thank the following individuals for their helpful comments on the manuscript: Michael Godkin, Marc Simmons, Joshua Singer, Bruce Webster, and Harris Faigel. I am sincerely grateful to Carol Curtis for her help in organizing, preparing and typing the manuscript. Her diligence and perseverance provided an important source of support. Thanks go to Lyn Riza as well, for helping with the figures. Finally, I am deeply grateful to Janice Quirk for her encouragement, patience and valuable assistance throughout the writing process.

CONTENTS

HOW TO LEARN AND TEACH
IN MEDICAL SCHOOL:
A LEARNER–CENTERED APPROACH

Part I

THE LEARNER

INTRODUCTION

In this section I will examine the ways in which medical students learn. I will describe the skills necessary to learn medicine and present exercises that students can use on their own, or within a course, to refine such skills. Mastery of these skills will enhance academic performance in medical school and residency and facilitate independent learning after formal training is finished. Medical education must undergo a paradigm shift in favor of the learner; a move away from predominately providing medical knowledge and skills toward teaching *how* to learn medicine. The need for such a shift has been recognized in the medical education literature for many years. Consider the wisdom and foresight of Willard Rappleye, head of the Commission on Medical Education for the Association of American Medical Colleges in 1932: " ... medicine is not taught by a faculty but is learned by one's own efforts, and the teaching is a question of stimulating each student instead of spoon-feeding him" (1933, p. 366).

Alan Gregg (1957), director of the Division of Medical Sciences of the Rockefeller Foundation, echoed this call for educational reform some twenty years later. He also began to characterize what was required:

> No school of medicine is worthy of the name that does not teach its students how to learn from experience as well as before experience, how to observe and reason wisely. ... He teaches best who shows his students how to learn: not what to think in 1953 but how to think and learn to think in that long stretch of days awaiting you till, let us say, the year 2000. (p. 50)

Those concerned with medical education had not been alone these years in calling for a new paradigm for learning and teaching. Theorists concerned with higher education in general also were calling for reform with emphasis on how to learn. (Rogers, 1969).

Medical educators gradually have come to recognize that providing

3

the necessary medical knowledge and skills is both an unrealistic task and insufficient preparation for future medical practice. It has now become increasingly apparent that medical education must focus on the *process* of learning to overcome the constraints associated with expected mastery of an increasingly excessive volume of medical content in a limited time, and the continuously shrinking half-life of medical knowledge and skills. This gradually unfolding enlightenment has been accompanied by a perceived need to view learning as a lifelong process for which medical students must be fully prepared. Smith states (1985):

> The true physician never graduates from medical school; he simply transfers from Harvard, Yale, the University of California at San Francisco, or wherever medical education has been started into a new and personalized "medical school." In this self-created school, he himself will be both faculty member and student. . . . It is imperative that we prepare our students for faculty membership in this second, intensely personal, and infinitely more important medical school, if, in fact, we know but how. (p. 108)

Unfortunately, we have not yet demonstrated that *we know but how.* Over the years, we have been told repeatedly that it is time to focus on skills which would enable learners to find solutions to complex problems and to ensure that they were prepared to continue learning independently throughout the practice of medicine. There has not been a commensurate unified process of developing medical school programs and strategies to meet these defined learning needs as there was in the early part of the twentieth century when the standardized medical school curriculum was adopted. We have not demonstrated a clear understanding of how *learning how to learn* can be implemented in the medical school curriculum.

Evidence that little progress in implementation has been made is reflected in the "highest priority" of the Proceedings of the Josiah Macy, Jr. Foundation, published more than three decades after Alan Gregg's proclamation, and more than a half century after Rappleye's report. This new priority states:

> Give more educational freedom to our medical student colleagues, trust them, and help them develop the skills they need to become self-reliant and effective lifelong learners. (Neufield, Bearpark & Winterton, 1989, p. 21)

As the perceived need for a new paradigm has strengthened in recent years, bold new initiatives which attempt to address some of the shortcomings have been implemented (Johnson & Shuster, 1992). Despite these noble efforts, we still lack a uniform notion of how medical students learn most effectively. What is needed for true reform is a clear and comprehensive picture of the skills required to learn medicine during medical school and beyond. This picture must be framed by solid learning theory.

It is the scientific approach itself which should guide our journey into the medical learning process. Eisenberg (1988) states:

> The fact is that medical education, far from being *too scientific,* suffers from too much emphasis on memorizing evanescent *facts* and too little on science as a way of framing questions and gathering evidence. (pp. 485–6)

Clearly, critical thinking, which includes the ability to solve problems, must be an important learning skill in the new paradigm.

The role of memorization, on the other hand, has been called into question. It has come to be associated with the term *rote* and has been overemphasized in the attempt to manage the *swelling* of content. Effective memorization, however, is essential to establishing a knowledge base.

The new paradigm for learning also would include the skill of self-evaluation. Barrows (1989) highlights the importance of this learning skill to clinical education:

> Students should be asked to assess their own performance with a patient, determine what they must learn to make a more satisfactory diagnosis and treatment plan, and identify the learning resource to employ. They should then be given the opportunity to dig out what they need to learn and come back to re-evaluate and improve their performance. (p. 49)

Critical thinking, memorizing, and self-evaluation are three examples of the skills necessary to learn in medical school. Barrows (1985) helps us to differentiate and integrate the levels of learning represented by each of these skills:

> . . . the medical students we educate must acquire (1) an essential body of knowledge, (2) the ability to use their knowledge effectively in the evaluation and care of their patients' health problems, and (3) the ability to extend or improve that knowledge and to provide appropriate care for future problems which they may face. (p. 3)

Using these three levels to frame our learner-centered approach we could describe the necessary learning skills as follows. First, to master a body of knowledge and to continually upgrade it, students must be able to effectively and efficiently read medical literature with comprehension and observe and record information presented verbally as well as visually. To store this information for use as knowledge, they must actively memorize this information with meaning and be able to access medical information now and in the future using new technologies. To use their knowledge in a clinical context with patients, students must acquire the basic learning skills of problem solving and communication. Finally, to be able to continue to learn independently after formal training, students must learn in medical school how to assess their own needs and to plan for, and evaluate, their own learning. The learning skills are summarized in Figure 1. Formal training in all of these required skills should begin on the first day of medical school.

Level	Task	Skills
I. Knowledge	Gathering, encoding and comprehending information	• Reading • Listening • Observing
II. Application	Using knowledge to gain new knowledge and solve problems	• Memorizing • Problem-Solving • Communicating
III. Self Instruction	Planning and implementing self-directed learning	• Analyzing needs • Developing goals • Identifying methods • Self-evaluating

Figure 1. Levels of learning with associated tasks and skills required for lifelong, learner-centered medical education.

This list of learning skills is not meant to be exclusive but rather to provide a foundation of *core skills* upon which the paradigm for learning in medical school will be built. They are the tools necessary to gather, encode, integrate, transfer, retrieve and use knowledge. As such, they are the foundation of *understanding* and *action.* The progression of skills from top to bottom represents an inverted hierarchy in which *higher order skills* incorporate elements of *lower order* skills. That is, gaining proficiency in skills at the top will help the learner to become proficient in the use of skills at the bottom. Conversely, students may experience difficulty becoming proficient in *new* learning skills if they haven't mastered *earlier* ones. The progressive order of skills reflects potential increased complexity and depth of learning gained from the use of each skill.

In sum, the evidence suggests that true curriculum reform in medical education is long overdue. The paucity of programmatic change which centers on learning and is grounded in learning theory suggests that we still lack a model for such reform. We have failed to specifically define the learning skills which are needed now more than ever and to outline a prescription for teaching them in the curriculum. In an effort to facilitate the development of a new paradigm for learning in medical school, the next four chapters will focus on the skills necessary to learn medicine. Guidelines for developing these skills will be presented for students, teachers, and those administrators responsible for developing and implementing medical school curricula. In addition, the importance of attending to learning differences among medical students will be demonstrated and discussed.

Chapter 1

GATHERING AND ENCODING INFORMATION
TO BUILD A KNOWLEDGE BASE

Three skills used to gather and encode information, that is, to gain knowledge, are reading, listening and observing. Each of these skills is essential to master the *core content* of medicine. In addition, these skills are antecedents of many *higher order* learning skills which are necessary to learn medicine in the clinical context.

READING SCIENTIFIC INFORMATION
FOR COMPREHENSION WITH SPEED

Harris and Sipay (1990) found that the average college student reads about 280 words per minute with excellent comprehension. They also report that superior college level readers read between 400–600 wpm with about seventy percent comprehension. They conclude that most readers can increase reading speed with comprehension.

According to Harris and Sipay (1990), average readers can increase their rate of reading by 25 to 50 percent without decreasing comprehension, and slow readers should be able to increase their reading rates by 50 to 100 percent using selected strategies and exercises. These findings are from studies which examine generic reading ability (e.g., English literature) and do not represent accurate estimates for reading scientific material which is much more condensed and complex and often includes new information.

To be a capable learner in medical school as well as after graduation, one must be able to read effectively and efficiently. Reading *effectively* means with comprehension and the ability to recall. Reading *efficiently* means reading effectively as quickly as possible. Reading should be an active rather than a passive process. The greatest barrier to effective and efficient reading for medical students is inattentiveness. Many of the techniques described below are directed toward increasing attention while reading scientific material.

9

Typically, reading a scientific passage for understanding requires using techniques which can significantly reduce reading rate at the expense of improving comprehension and recall. These techniques (e.g., note-making) help the reader accurately assess the meaning assigned by the writer and then to incorporate this meaning into a personal frame of reference which will aid future recall and use. The effective reader must employ such strategies which facilitate attention, aid interpretation, and ultimately enhance comprehension of meaning.

Readers in medical school should be able to vary their approaches to reading depending upon the type of material to be read (e.g., biochemistry textbook vs. prepared course handout) and the goal of reading (preview vs. review vs. assimilation of new material). This flexibility of reading behavior, depending upon the goals and type of material, characterizes effective reading. With the extremely high and often unrealistic reading demands of medical school, it is important to be efficient as well as flexible in one's approach.

To be flexible, active, and to establish meaning are the goals of effective and efficient reading. The following steps will help you to achieve these goals. You should assess your own reading needs in relation to each of these steps and use the strategies described to increase your reading skills. Faculty should encourage students to use these steps and develop their curricula with them in mind (e.g., handouts should have clear, meaningful headings and subheadings for preview).

Step 1: Plan

Taylor (1992) found that the time necessary to complete *required* readings for second-year students at one medical school totaled sixty-two hours per week. For the dedicated medical student this leaves little time for eating, sleeping and going to class. With such unrealistic expectations for reading, many students who might do well otherwise would not perform satisfactorily if they attempt to read everything. Planning begins with prioritizing the importance of *all* readings, including those that are required, and realizing that not all will be read. Once you have decided what to read, define your purpose and decide how much you will read in the time you have allotted. If your purpose is to assimilate new information, as opposed to reviewing previously read material, then you will require more time and will employ different techniques. Having specific goals (e.g., read a new twenty-page biochemistry handout in two hours) will direct your reading activity by increasing your motivation to finish.

Be *realistic* in deciding how much you can read, and try to achieve your goal. It may take practice to identify your volume and attention limits, and they will vary with each course and the type of, and your familiarity with, the material (e.g., new chapter, previously read handout). It is important to limit the time you spend reading one topic during one sitting to afford maximum concentration. Ideally, schedule reading in blocks of three or less hours for each subject and try to read for detail and understanding during peak concentration times (e.g., early morning). Use shorter amounts of time for review and reinforcing long-term memorization (see memorization below).

Step 2: Preview for Meaning

Before you begin to read for detail and understanding, preview the material to be read during your available block of time. This involves skimming through the section headings, subheadings, and, if time permits, the first and last sentences of each paragraph to form a picture of the whole and its parts. Research has demonstrated that paying close attention to headings will result in significant positive gain on tests of scientific readings (Brooks et al., 1983). Previewing written material includes both attending to the visual cues (e.g., headings) and engaging in the mental exercise of anticipating or predicting the content.

The process of anticipating content serves two purposes. First, it is the initial step in establishing personal meaning for the written material by using your own words. As you will see, establishing personal meaning greatly enhances retention and recall (e.g., during examinations or application of knowledge). Second, it will serve as a foundation from which to reassess or check meaning during focused reading. Reassessment is an active learning process which holds attention and will almost always help create a valid interpretation of the author's meaning.

Attending to the visual cues represented by the headings helps the reader define a context (viz., the whole) which helps find meaning in each part. Often the meaning of the part one is reading (e.g., irreversible enzyme inhibition) becomes clear only when you already are familiar with the broader context, specific information, or examples (e.g., pennicilloyl-enzyme with transpeptidase) to be presented later in the text.

Consider another example. If I am required to read a handout entitled aerobic gram positive bacilli and closely related microorganisms, it would help to know that both gram-positive and gram-negative, cocci and bacilli, will be described and differentiated by aerobic and anaerobic. As I read about non-branching and branching (viz., connecting) characteristics of aerobic, gram-positive bacilli, I begin to realize from my preview that they are characteristics of both anaerobic and aerobic non-spore-forming bacilli. These early associations not only enhance reading comprehension by adding meaning but will aid later memorization by providing common words (non-branching, branching) and visual cues to link ideas and to organize thoughts.

Once you have previewed a selected passage, section, or handout, be prepared to read in a focused manner and then to re-read for review at a later time. In most instances, an appropriate reading strategy would include these three steps: preview, focused reading, and review. Each step is essential to efficient and effective reading and requires a different amount of time and the use of specific strategies. Focused reading is the centerpiece of reading activity and requires the most time to accomplish.

Step 3: Focused Reading

Mindful Note-Taking

Research has demonstrated that although underlining is more effective than just reading, writing notes during reading leads to significantly greater comprehension, as assessed on performance tests, than either underlining or simply reading alone (Annis & Davis, 1978). However, what you write will determine whether this activity enhances reading comprehension or is simply a *passive* exercise in futility.

Writing verbatim and overwriting while reading, are passive and can be a waste of time. Focus writing on *your thoughts,* make connections between concepts, jot details that increase understanding. Write your thoughts in your own words. Be selective. Write only those things that you feel are important. There may be whole sections where no writing is necessary. Either you know the material well enough or it is not so important. Challenge yourself to understand by *interpreting* and *summarizing.* If you do not write as you read, try it. Research has demonstrated that using strategies which you might *not* normally choose can lead to improved learning performance. This suggests that the use of new strategies may increase attention, thereby increasing comprehension of what is read.

During focused reading, write descriptors, concepts and details in the margins while you read. Writing is an indispensable part of focused reading of science. Descriptors are terms that convey special meaning to a body of material. For example, in anatomy, nerve descriptors would include somatic, autonomic, cranial, spinal, lumbar, sacral, etc. Bone descriptors would include short, long, flat, irregular, etc. In physiology, enzyme descriptors include saturation, selectivity, competition, etc. Develop your own personal set of descriptors for each unit of each class and use them to organize your thoughts while you read. Write and summarize concepts and make interpretations using abbreviations when necessary.

Develop a system for representing relationships among details, concepts, and ideas in your notes. Draw your own simple figures and *maps* to represent relationships among concepts and details as you read. Use an outline format with indentations to show how details describe or relate to a specific concept. As you write, compare and contrast in your mind what you read with what you anticipated the section would be about. Some examples of margin notes are provided. Read the following excerpt on DNA from Stryer (1988). Figure 2 presents an example of how, in your notes, to visually represent or *diagram* the relationships important for understanding DNA from reading this excerpt.

DNA is a polymer of deoxyribonucleotide units. A *nucleotide* consists of a nitrogenous base, a sugar, and one or more phosphate groups. The sugar in a deoxyribonucleotide is *deoxyribose.* The *deoxy* prefix indicates that this sugar lacks an oxygen atom that is present in ribose, the parent compound. The nitrogenous base is a derivative of *purine* or pyrimidine.

In a deoxyribonucleotide, the C-1 carbon atom of deoxyribose is bonded to N-1 of a pyrimidine or N-9 of a purine. The configuration of this N-glycosidic linkage is β (the base lies above the plane of the sugar ring). A *nucleoside* consists of a purine or pyrimidine base bonded to a sugar. The four *nucleoside units in DNA* are called *deoxyadenosine, deoxyguanosine, deoxythymidine,* and *deoxycytidine.* A *nucleotide* is a phosphate ester of a nucleoside. The most common site of esterification in naturally occurring nucleotides is the hydroxyl group attached to C-5 of the sugar. Such a compound is called a *nucleoside 5-phosphate* or a 5'-nucleotide. For example, deoxyadenosine 5'-triphosphate (dATP) is an activated precursor in the synthesis of DNA. A primed number denotes an atom of the sugar, whereas an unprimed number denotes an atom of the purine or pyrimidine ring. The prefix *d* in dATP indicates that the

Deoxyribonucleotide

Components

Unit	bond			bond	Unit
		Base (nitrogenous)	(variable)		
Nucleoside					**Nucleotide**
• deoxyadenosine • deoxyguanosine • deoxythymidine • deoxycytidine	⌐N-9 ⌐N-1	purines 　• adenine (A) 　• guanine (G) pyrimidines 　• thymine (T) 　• cytosine (C)			• deoxyadenylate • deoxyguanylate • deoxycytidylate • deoxythymidylate
	C-1	sugar (deoxyribose)	– – –	C-5	'nucleoside 5 phosphate'
		Phosphodiester bridge			
					– –(backbone)
		sugar (deoxyribose)	_ _ _		

Figure 2. Notes on DNA relationships distilled from a textbook (Stryer, 1988).

sugar is deoxyribose to distinguish this compound from ATP, in which the sugar is ribose.

The *backbone* of DNA, which is invariant throughout the molecule, consists of deoxyriboses linked to phosphate groups. Specifically, the 3'-hydroxyl of the sugar moiety of one deoxyribonucleotide is joined to the 5'-hydroxyl of the adjacent sugar by a phosphodiester bridge. The *variable part* of DNA is its *sequence of four kinds of bases (A, G, C, and T)*. The corresponding nucleotide units are called *deoxyadenylate, deoxyguanylate, deoxycytidylate,* and *deoxythymidylate.*

At the end of a section, write a brief statement or create a diagram to represent your understanding of the material. At the end of a chapter write a more detailed summary in your own words from immediate recall. These *activities* help to synthesize your thoughts as well as maintain your attention and enhance understanding. When reading particularly dense material (viz., many details), you may want to demonstrate more often, using diagrams, the relationships among component parts of a whole, or similarities and differences among subtopics or concepts.

Although this can be *labor intensive* and will slow your reading rate, it will enhance your comprehension and ultimately facilitate your recall. The following flow diagram (Figure 3) was constructed while reading a handout on bacteria and closely related organisms.

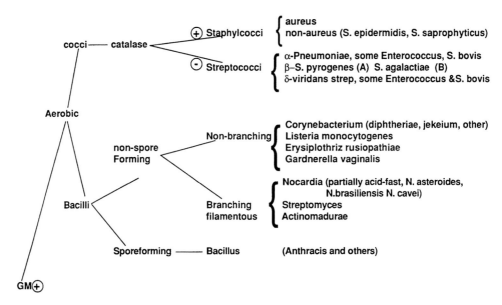

Figure 3. Flow diagram based on a handout concerning bacteria and closely related microorganisms.

Read for Details and Understanding

Read phrases; don't read word by word. Get into a rhythm. Meaning and understanding will be established more quickly. This rhythm will vary with the complexity of, and your familiarity with, the material. If you are fully concentrating you should be able to anticipate the next words and sentences you are about to read. You will feel the continuity of meaning (viz., understanding) from one phrase, one sentence, and even one paragraph to the next. This contrasts with reading rote (word by word) which fragments meaning and reduces understanding and attention.

This reading technique takes practice to perfect and courage to use. It often means recognizing and reducing internalized anxiety associated with a fear that one is *missing something* if every word is not read. Early educational experiences which include reading orally in class are the basis of our only formal model of reading. Most often during these oral reading exercises the educational objectives, which are defined by the teacher, are to improve *word* pronunciation and enhance *word* recognition. Reading phrases for meaning and understanding is not usually part of our early learning experiences.

As you read, don't become focused on the meaning of individual words
in the sentence but feel confident that short-term memory and concentration will carry you through until broader and *more relevant* understanding is achieved later in the sentence, or in some instances, in the paragraph. The goal is to ascertain an essential understanding of the written series of words, which is greater than the sum of its parts. Not all of the words in the series are of equal importance to this goal. Key words are an essential ingredient of meaning units or phrases. Consider the following example from a course handout on the neuromuscular junction (NMJ):

> We may propose the following explanation of *postsynaptic events,* whether at the NMJ or elsewhere: The *transmitter interacts* with *receptors* in the *postsynaptic membrane* to *alter* the *membrane's permeability or conductance* for *one or more ions. Local currents* are thereby *generated* in the *region of synapse* in the *postsynaptic neuron or muscle fiber.* These local currents may have either an *excitatory* or *inhibitory* effect. If they *drive* the *membrane* potential (V_m) toward threshold as the neuromuscular junction, they are *excitatory.* If they *prevent V_m from moving toward threshold,* they are *inhibitory;* that is, they tend to prevent the generation of an action potential in the postsynaptic structure.

It seems quite clear from this example that if one actively searches for the meaningful words in a paragraph, then reading becomes both more efficient and effective. Less meaningful connecting words and repetitious statements can be ignored. At the same time the search process itself increases attention, thereby enhancing understanding and ultimately recall. Having to interrupt concentration on the *larger* meaning of sentences and paragraphs, to focus on less meaningful words, also will dramatically reduce reading rate.

As you read to understand with efficiency, move quickly through sentences finding essential meaning from the sums of key words, or *meaning units.* If after substantial practice you experience difficulty reading this way, you may have a word-recognition problem and need to improve your vocabulary (see Chapter 5). A common symptom of this problem is fixating on less familiar words and having to re-read sentences three or more times to establish meaning (Harris & Sipay, 1990).

If you experience fixations which primarily focus on medical terminology, keep a *running glossary* of these terms for each course and study it. Be sure to concentrate on pronunciation as you read. Don't read *through* key words, without pronouncing them. Quite often our tendency is to do this, especially those which are new. This not only will perpetuate fixations of the same word the next time it is encountered but also will diminish recognition (and ultimately recall). If you fixate primarily on lay terms, you may need to review basic vocabulary texts (e.g., Miller, 1967) or work with a reading specialist (see Chapter 5).

One exercise you can use to enhance the speed and accuracy of word recognition while at the same time *improving memory* of course material is to develop (from your running glossary) a series of flash cards with vocabulary words and phrases common to your readings yet new to your vocabulary. On each card, print the word and indicate the pronunciation on one side, and define it on the other side. Continue to add to this series of cards as the course progresses.

To enhance word recognition for purposes of increasing reading rate with comprehension, move as quickly as possible through the series of cards, looking only at the sides with the vocabulary word. During this exercise (as opposed to focusing on memory), study the definition sides of the cards *only* if you don't recognize the word's meaning. Using this flash card technique when reading new and unfamiliar material will increase word recognition and improve your reading rate.

Another exercise for improving your ability to read in meaning units is to use slashes or a highlighter to identify these units and the key words in a reading passage. Immediately after you apply this technique, re-read the passage or section, focusing only on the identified meaning units and key words. This will reinforce reading in phrases for meaning.

There is danger in highlighting too much. Often students who highlight too much are not focusing on meaning units and key words but rather use the highlighter as a substitute for their finger to keep their place, to maintain attention, and/or to provide a sense of security (viz., if it's all in yellow, then it's in my brain). Practice highlighting less by learning to focus on details and key words and ultimately highlighting only those meaning units and key words *which you don't know.* This will help you make reading a less passive process. As you continue to use this exercise, it becomes easier to read in meaning units during focused reading and re-reading will be unnecessary.

Goal-Directed Reading

During reading, continually remind yourself of your goal: to establish specific meaning and gain understanding for the purpose of recall. Don't waste time simply reading to finish. If we do not continually remind ourselves of our goals, often our minds wander or we focus on meaning which is not central to our purpose. For example, as we read a case presentation on a patient with a productive cough who smokes cigarettes, our goal may be to learn how to characterize the cough or how to introduce smoking cessation. Sometimes there are multiple goals to be defined.

One exercise designed to reinforce this strategy may seem artificial at first. Before you begin your next reading assignment, set your alarm clock or watch alarm for five minutes. When the alarm sounds, assess the amount of time during the five-minute interval that you were actually concentrating on meaning and understanding for purposes of later recall. Reset the alarm, refocus on your goal, and begin again. Continue this exercise until you are comfortable that most of the time that you are reading during this session you are concentrating on your goal for the purpose of recall. Get a good feel for goal-directed reading so that you begin to associate it with all of your science reading. Continue to use this exercise until you internalize the technique of goal-directed reading and then use the exercise periodically thereafter to reinforce the concept and skill.

The Mechanics of Reading

Maintain steady and paced eye movement across and down the page. It is important to avoid regressions or backward eye movements in reading (Harris & Sipay, 1990). This is perhaps the most mechanical aspect of reading yet one which we rarely, if ever, attend to. It is important to move forward to the next line rather than repeating the line or even regressing back to the previous line. In addition, the reader must not *fall off* the end of a line or *reach beyond* the beginning of the next line. Try to maintain your focus in the middle of a page or column as you sweep through phrases and key words down the page. Return sweeps should be a single quick diagonal movement from the end of one line to the beginning of the next (Harris & Sipay, 1990).

If you find that you do regress, use Figure 4 to create a full-page chart for practicing steady and paced eye movement. As you advance in your practice of this skill, you can replace the X's and O's with words and phrases like those found in the paragraph on the neuromuscular junction above. Consciously exaggerate the sweep as you read. It should become more natural with practice.

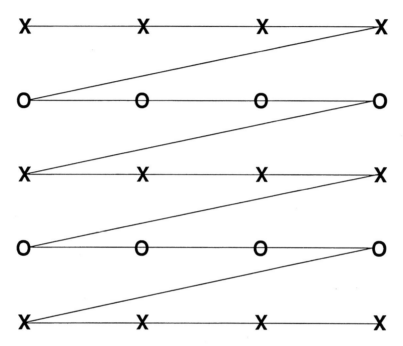

Figure 4. Cross-line exercise for improving eye coordination. (Courtesy of Harris and Sippay, 1990, p. 646.)

Step 4: Review

Review what you previously read before the exam. Research has demonstrated that reading for review can significantly improve performance on multiple-choice exams. Annis and Davis (1977) state: "Apparently review strengthens the direct or mediated linkage between the material previously encoded during the study period and the responses needed for success on a multiple-choice test" (p. 178).

This step more closely approximates the preview step than focused reading. You should concentrate on headings, subheadings, topic sentences, notes and figures in the margins, and highlighted meaning units. It is extremely important during this step not to be distracted by focusing on what you already know. Students do this too often just as they do with highlighting. Once again, the purpose is to recall *personal meaning* assigned to the author's words and not to rehash old meaning nor to establish new meaning (unless absolutely necessary). This distinction of purpose is very important and should guide your reading activity during review.

It is the student's responsibility to follow these steps and use these techniques to read and master course material and to prepare for lifelong independent learning. You must recognize that even with the development and use of these important reading strategies, *your* reading ability will differ from other medical students. These strategies will maximize your potential, but ultimately you will be limited by your capacity to comprehend and your speed to process what you read, as well as your ability to regulate eye movements, your interest in the material, etc.

Faculty and curriculum coordinators must answer the question: *What is the basic competency level in reading speed and comprehension we expect of our medical students in our course?* Once they have the answer, they must teach to, as well as evaluate at, that level. Those students who are more competent in this skill area will read more effectively and efficiently than the average student. Those students who do not achieve this basic competency level will not be able to read and understand all of the course material nor complete the exams in as timely a fashion.

As previously noted, one problem with medical education in its current form is that the amount of required readings in medical school is unrealistic. It is the course and clerkship coordinator's responsibility to establish reading requirements which are realistic (viz., recognizing that students take more than one course at a time) and pertinent to training medical students (not graduate students in a basic science discipline nor residents in a medical specialty). During the preclinical years, students should not be required to read more than five to seven hours per week in any one course. Required reading material ultimately must be essential to application (critical thinking, communication and problem solving) and must be clearly and concisely presented. Depth of the material should reflect the student's chosen profession (medicine) and level of training. Evaluation of knowledge gained through reading should stress the meaning of the material and not recall or recognition of *less* meaningful facts. Ample time should be offered for all students to complete their examinations. Faculty must consider these criteria for selecting their required readings and developing their course examinations if they are to meet the reading needs of their students.

If a student shows signs of potential reading difficulty, it is the course coordinator's responsibility to identify resources and to provide assistance by reasonably accommodating to the learner's needs. For example, some students may need more time on exams than others, or may need to be in a separate room where they can vocalize written test questions and their answers without distracting other students. In many instances, the ultimate goal is to integrate students into timed and group test-taking conditions. However, if these conditions result in inaccurate or invalid assessment of performance for some students, then the conditions should be redefined for these students. This *flexibility* characterizes a learner-centered approach to medical education. Our experience has demonstrated that accommodating to individual reading needs during examinations can result in dramatic increases in academic performance.

The importance of reading scientific material for comprehension with speed should be introduced on the first day of medical school and formally taught within the context of medical school. Required readings in each course could provide the raw material for this early instruction. Faculty can devise their own examples like the ones cited in this chapter to illustrate the principles and strategies of effective and efficient reading. Students would gain relevant medical knowledge at the same time that they are learning to apply reading strategies. Subsequent courses should revisit these reading strategies with teaching sessions devoted to reinforcing them within the context of the new course content. In addition, faculty in all courses should ensure that course material is consistent with the principles of good reading (e.g., handouts are well organized, requirements are realistic). A strong commitment by faculty will be necessary to ensure that medical students learn to read scientific material effectively, and that reading is a profitable and enjoyable learning experience.

Students who experience reading problems should be offered the opportunity to receive intensive individual tutoring in reading (see Chapter 5 for definition and description). This would include a student whose academic performance is consistently inhibited by poor comprehension, speed, or vocabulary, as well as a student with more severe reading disability (e.g., diagnosed dyslexia). Neglecting to help students develop reading skills not only decreases what they learn during medical school but also lessens their chances of performing optimally as more independent learners during residency and later during practice.

LISTENING AND TAKING NOTES

In addition to reading, a second skill used extensively in medical school to gather and encode information is listening and taking notes. It is used to facilitate learning during lectures, labs, discussion groups and even during interactions with patients. It may be operationally defined as *the ability to summarize in writing what is presented orally in order to enhance understanding* and *facilitate recall.*

The steps and the strategies which define this skill are similar to those involved in reading. The underlying objectives are to add personal meaning to the content presented thus enhancing understanding and maintaining attention. Students should follow these steps and practice these strategies to gather and encode material which is presented orally.

Step 1: Preview

Preview any written material that is relevant to the presentation, particularly handouts which are distributed by the teacher prior to the class. You should *briefly* scan the written material to acquire familiarity with the topics and terms to be covered. Headings and subheadings should be noted, and unfamiliar words and terms should be highlighted and defined (using reference material) in the margins. Previewing will provide a deeper understanding of the parts in relation to the whole and improve word recognition when presented orally. This will free you from trying to establish understanding with significant gaps in meaning during the lecture.

Step 2: Focused Listening

Organizing Your Notes

During the presentation concentrate on understanding and organize what you write by showing the relationships among the pieces of information presented. An indented format (Willey & Jarecky, 1976) may be helpful in this regard. Start with a topic, list the explanatory and descriptive details and include the details about the details. Consider the following example in Figure 5, constructed from the same handout on bacteria and closely related organisms.

Several other strategies will enhance the effectiveness and the efficiency of your listening and note-taking. First, it is important to remem-

I. **Aerobic gram positive Cocci**

  A. **Staphylocci (clusters, catalase positive)**

    1. **Staphylococcus aureus**

    2. **Non-aureus staphylococci**

      a. **S. epidermidis**
      b. **S. saprophyticus**
      c. **Nine other species**

  B. **Streptococci (pairs and chains, catalase negative)**

    1. **Alpha hemolytic streptococci**

      a. **Streptococcus pneumoniae**
      b. **Viridans streptococci (eight species)**
      c. **Enterococcus species (three)**
      d. **Streptococcus bovis**

    2. **Beta hemolytic streptococci**

      a. **Group A (S. pyogenes)**
      b. **Group B (S. agalactiae)**
      c. **Group C, F and G**

    3. **Gamma hemolytic streptococci--some strains of viridans strep, Enterococcus and S. bovis**

II. **Aerobic gram positive bacilli (non-spore forming)**

  A. **Non-branching**

    1. **Corynebacterium**

      a. **Corynebacterium diphtheriae**
      b. **Corynebacterium jekeium**
      c. **Numerous other species (the aerobic diphtheroids)**

    2. **Listeria monocytogenes**

    3. **Erysiplothrix rusiopathiae**

    4. **Gardnerella vaginalis**

  B. **Branching, filamentous**

    1. **Nocardia (partially acid-fast)**

      a. **N. asteroides**
      b. **N. brasiliensis**
      c. **N. cavei**

    2. **Streptomyces species**

    3. **Actinomadurae species**

III. **Aerobic gram positive bacilli (spore-forming)**

  A. **Bacillus**
    1. **Bacillus anthracis**
    2. **Numerous other species**

Figure 5. Indented format based on handout concerning bacteria and closely related microorganisms.

ber that listening differs from reading in that information is gathered at *someone else's* pace. It is important to be prepared for receiving information that is transmitted rapidly. Develop abbreviations and symbols for common, and course-specific, words and use them consistently throughout all your course notes. Figure 6 presents some examples of symbols and abbreviations for common words and phrases in medicine. It is important to develop your own abbreviations for words and groups of words used often in a single course. Whenever possible, write your notes from your own thoughts using your own words and symbols. Not only will this improve the efficiency of data gathering, it will add meaning to the information by initiating the encoding process and will help maintain your attention during listening.

Active Listening

During encoding, remember to concentrate on listening first, then on writing. This will give you an opportunity to *translate* what you hear into your own thoughts and feelings. Write *meaning units* and not simply words. During this process, writing is secondary to listening. Often students fail to initially listen and translate and simply try to write verbatim what they hear. In this regard, attending lecture (or interacting with a patient) becomes a passive process akin to reading without comprehension. Encoding often is neglected by students during lectures, thus leading one medical educator to say that: "A lecture [is] a process by which information is transferred from the notes of the lecturer to the notes of the student without going through the minds of either" (Simpson, 1972, p. 98).

During lecture, don't dwell on information or concepts that you don't completely understand. Incorporate a mechanism into your note-taking that allows you to quickly identify and remediate incomplete understanding at a later time. This will allow you to more fully concentrate on what the presenter is saying to you now. For example, if you are right-handed, take notes during lecture only on the right-side pages in your notebook. Leave the left-side pages blank so you can later enter information from other sources (e.g., handouts, textbooks) that answers questions and contributes to understanding the lecture notes.

As you listen and write, use abbreviations (e.g., supr ster $\downarrow$ fibrobl), and draw diagrams and figures as often as possible to describe part-whole relationships or to represent directionality in means-ends processes. These drawings can be accomplished quickly during the lecture to increase

↓	decrease	+	excess
↑	increase	-	deficient
>	greater than	**Dx**	diagnosis
<	less than	**c/o**	complained of
♂	male	**Hx**	history
♀	female	**(L)**	left
s&s	signs & symptoms	**(R)**	right
L→R	left to right	†	death
P	parent	∞	infinite
α	alpha	β	beta
Ab	antibody	**ANS**	autonomic nervous system
ABC	abbreviated blood count	**ABEP**	auditory brain stem--evoked potentials
ACLR	anterior cruciate ligament repair	**BACT**	bacteria
BP	blood pressure	**CMV**	cytomegalovirus
CIBD	chronic inflammatory bowel disease	**CNDC**	chronic nonspecific diarrhea of childhood
CNS	central nervous disease	**HBV**	hepatitis B virus
HCVD	hypertensive cardiovascular disease	**HSV**	herpes simples virus
Γ	gamma	**LRQ**	lower right quadrant
MAO	monoamine oxidase	**PLV**	posterior left ventricular
NADP	oxidixed nicotinamide adenine dinucleotide phosphate	**TPVR**	total peripheral vascular resistance
STIs	systolic time intervals	**1°**	primary
→	leads to	**2°**	secondary
		3°	tertiary

Figure 6. Common symbols and abbreviations in medicine. (Entries from Bhushan et al., 1993, and Davis, 1990.)

understanding and to facilitate verbal following. In keeping with your reading strategy, these drawings should be crude and use word abbreviations and rough approximations of shapes. They can be refined, if necessary, after class. Consider the following simple diagram (Figure 7) representing intercellular electrical communication.

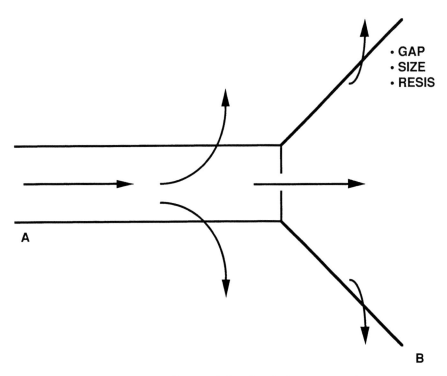

Figure 7. Diagram of intracellular electrical communication.

This diagram enhances later recall of details from the lecture such as: (1) current will flow rather than be shunted away if the gap is obliterated; (2) provided that resistance of the membrane where the cells are in contact is much lower than for the rest of the membrane in cell A; and (3) size of the junction must be reasonable in relation to the size of the cells.

Learning these strategies takes time and practice. It is a good idea to practice them on class notes already taken or on audiotapes or videotapes of previous lectures.

Step 3: Review

As soon as possible after class, spend fifteen to twenty minutes reviewing your class notes for inconsistencies, questions to be answered, incomplete thoughts or meaning, and inaccuracies. Just as in reading, complete understanding of material presented in a lecture often doesn't occur until the end (either of a chapter or a lecture). It is important to identify gaps, to complete lines of thought, and to correct inaccuracies while the information is fresh in your mind. Just as in review of reading, it is important to *not* focus on what you know. This early review completes the encoding process and represents the first step toward internalizing or memorizing the new information.

OBSERVING THE PATIENT AND THE ENVIRONMENT

Observation involves the use of strategies which enable the student to gather and encode information during demonstrations and labs and ultimately to learn about the patient and his/her problem. With respect to the latter, observational skills enable the physician to develop an accurate description of physical, personal, and interpersonal characteristics of the patient and the environment. These characteristics of the patient and environment are extremely important sources of information which, when combined with knowledge, skills and feelings obtained from other sources (e.g., from reading and listening described above, or from questioning described under communication skills below) will be used in clinical problem solving.

Observational skills required to learn medicine include visual-spatial, tactile and interpersonal perceptual skills. The Special Advisory Panel on Technical Standards for Medical School Admission (AAMC, 1978) identifies observation as one of five skill areas required for successful completion of the M.D. degree. They define this learning skill as "the ability to observe demonstrations and experiments in the basic sciences," and later, under communication, "the ability to observe patients . . . to describe changes in mood, activity, and posture, and perceive nonverbal communications." Although strategies involved in observing the physical and interpersonal environments share many similarities, there are also distinctive features of each which must be recognized and learned.

Development of observational skills will enable you to learn from your laboratories, patients and from colleagues. You should practice the skills individually or with tutors using the recommended exercises.

Spatial-Perceptual Learning Skills

Spatial-perceptual skills are defined by Rochford (1985) as:

> ... the ability to perceive, retain and recognize (or reproduce) three-dimensional objects in their correct proportions when they are rotated in space, translated, juxtaposed, projected, sectioned, re-assembled, inverted, re-oriented or verbally described. (p. 14)

Spatial perceptual skills share a close association with other basic learning skills which are used to gather and encode data. Once again, an essential strategy is to establish personal meaning which enhances understanding of the information being gathered. Especially in perception, establishing meaning often involves using prior knowledge to define the relevance, function, or relationship of the whole to other objects. In this connection, Olson and Bialystok (1983) state: "What we know — our expectancies and our interpretations in conjunction with the sensory display determine what we perceive" (p. 5).

In addition to relying on what we know, spatial perception involves developing a *structural description* of the whole being perceived, using its parts and the relationships among them (Olson & Bailystok, 1983). Structural descriptions include the use of such concepts as size, shape, location, distance, color, height, weight, depth, etc. For example, one's perception of a red blood cell might be: one section is red, the other is clear (e.g., *the large section was red, the smaller section clear*). In addition, a structural description can include information about the relationship or interactions among such features (e.g., size by color) and the relationship among parts or the parts to the whole. The latter might include descriptors like *beside one another* or *extending out from one side*, etc. Consider the following description of what was observed during a lab demonstration in organ biology (Figure 8):

Scanning EM of splenic sinuses: Notice erythrocytes (Er) *migrating between* endothelial cells (EC). The *interior* of the splenic sinus is shown in Figures 2 (human) and 3 (rat). The *long* axis of the endothelial cells *parallels* that of the sinus.

Figure 8. Structuralist view of a lab demonstration.

Perception must account for both the relationships among parts and characteristics of the whole. Palmer (1977) uses the description of a square to exemplify these two distinct perspectives which must be integrated. The *structuralist* position would view the square as a collection of four lines of equal length joined at the ends to make right angles. The *gestalt* position would focus on the whole, as well as the attributes of closedness and area, which convey functional meaning.

As a medical student you must develop observational skills related to these two perspectives. Knowing and practicing them will enhance academic performance in those courses and rotations which emphasize their learning value (e.g., anatomy, pathology, surgery), and ultimately improve patient care. Consider these two perspectives represented in the following observations of the GI tract (Figure 9): Thorough familiarity and practice with the full range of descriptors, from both a structuralist and a gestalt perspective, will help develop the ability to build descriptions and strengthen perception.

Structural descriptions can be organized to ensure that all important features and part-whole relations are included. Figure 10 presents a list of important structural descriptors used to perceive objects in medicine.

Palmer (1977) and Gibson (1969) offer important guidance in learning how to expand our perception by considering the parts *in relation* to the whole. Palmer (1977) states that an entire network of parts which constitute the object being observed, is dominated by a structural network called a *schema.* He states: "The schema integrates all of the information known about the scene, object, or part into a systematic framework used during perceptual processing" (p. 444). When considering the whole, it is important to view it in terms of function as well as integration of parts.

Within the schema *simpler* elements are *selectively* grouped into higher-order parts. We do this selectively because one couldn't possibly consider all reasons for grouping. Rather, grouping is based upon such personal meaning issues as perceived importance, utility, familiarity, etc. Some of these reasons for grouping are more *commonly accepted* than others (Palmer's concept of "goodness of parts"). Some may be very situation or discipline specific (viz., relate to one course more than another). Learners often, through force of habit and to the detriment of learning, consider *only one* criterion for grouping and often that criterion is familiarity. Perception is greatly enhanced when we challenge ourselves to perceive alternative groupings. Consider the following view of the skull: Structurally, this superior view can be perceived as a whole

MUCOSA

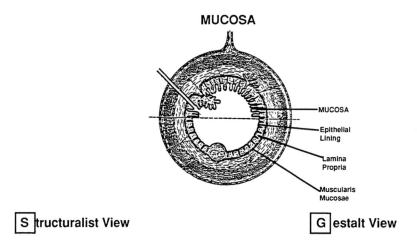

S tructuralist View   **G** estalt View

1. innermost layer
   (closest to lumen)

2. composed of *epithelium*,
   an underlying loose
   connective tissue layer,
   the *lamina propria*, and a
   smooth muscle layer, the
   muscularis mucosae.

The mucosa allows
the tract to 'communicate'
with the outside world.'
It serves as the conduit
for absorption.

Figure 9. Structuralist and Gestalt view of the GI tract (mucosa).

which is divided into four discrete sections: frontal, occipital, right and left. Alternatively, it may be perceived as a collection of three bones, three sutures, two intersections and two *other* features.

In terms of the *whole* (gestalt) it is uniquely suited to protect the brain of the growing human. The sutures allow for expansion of the protective plate during growth. The parietal bones form the *roof* and *walls* of the skull, and the foramen is a passage for vessels and nerves.

As learners we must challenge ourselves to gain a perspective of the whole (which includes the relationships among parts as well as function) and to view the relationships among the parts in new and different ways. We can call this strategy *perspective-taking*.

Gibson (1969) helps us to understand perception by calling our attention to the importance of discriminating. Accordingly, the development of perceptual abilities is reflected in an increased capacity to process "stimulus information that allows the perceiver to discriminate between

Category	Descriptors
size	massive, limited
shape/appearance	spiral, elongated
proximity	remote, proximal
position	posterior, bilateral, anterior
number	all, none, additional
movement	migrate laterally, radiate
amount	entire, partial
location	mid-brain, midline

Figure 10. Examples of structural descriptors. (Excerpted from Olson and Bailystock, 1983, p. 150.)

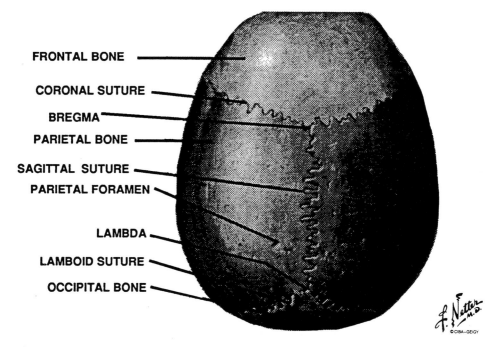

Figure 11. Superior view of skull. (Courtesy of Netter, 1989.) Copyright 1989, CIBA–GEIGY Corporation. Reprinted with permission from the Atlas of Human Anatomy, illustrated by Frank H. Netter, M.D. All rights reserved.

similar things which he did not initially distinguish" (Flavell, 1977, p. 154). I would suggest that our perception is enhanced by comparing characteristics, both similar and different, of focal objects we observe with those we recall. Comparing unfamiliar objects to those with which we are familiar expedites perception by giving us clues as to how parts might relate to the whole and also about function. This is a strategy that can be practiced and should be incorporated into all of your perceptual tasks.

It is clear that establishing perceptual meaning relies on your previous knowledge and your ability to draw comparisons. It is the meaning which drives the development of structural descriptions by serving as the criterion for selecting and grouping features and defining functional relations (Olson & Bailystok, 1983). Although one *cannot practice* previous knowledge, certainly one's skill at drawing comparisons based on available cues and knowledge can be practiced.

Suppose we are familiar with the esophagus and our task is to *learn* the colon. We would begin by perceiving both parts in relation to the whole digestive tube. We could then compare the new object (colon) with the more familiar object (esophagus), in terms of similarities and differences in functional and structural characteristics. How would you describe similarities and differences in functional and structural characteristics of the colon and the esophagus?

One other important aspect of perception involves the relation between you, the observer, and the object being observed. This is often referred to as the perceptual *orientation*. Gaining proficiency in perceptual orientation is an extremely important strategy in medical learning and practice.

Often in medical education, objects (e.g., organs, bones) which were learned one way (viz., from one view or vantage point) are presented for inspection from another orientation (e.g., during anatomy labs, practical exams, slide presentations). They are rotated in space. One strategy for enhancing perceptual ability to retrieve knowledge originally from another view is to initially study objects from both the perspective in which they are presented and from other *imaginary* perspectives. This involves rotating the object in your mind as you study it and attempting to discern what the object would look like from other vantage points. Short of physically manipulating the object, this is the most active strategy for increasing perceptual orientation.

A strategy which uses similar techniques but is accomplished *post hoc* during recall is to rotate the newly presented object in imaginary space back to its *original* position (initially presented and learned) through successive small increments. This technique has been suggested as an aid to recall by Just and Carpenter (1976).

The strategies for enhancing perceptual orientation demand a systematic approach to viewing the object. Olson and Bailystok (1983) define positional dimensions and axes which are helpful in perceiving orientation and rotation.

Type	Characteristics	Rotation	Invariant dimension	Variable dimensions
lateral	depth around horizontal axis	top toward / top away	left/right	top bottom
vertical	depth around vertical axis	right toward/ right away	top/bottom	front/back left/right
frontal	plane rotation	clockwise/ counterclock- wise 'spin'	front/back	top/bottom left/right

Figure 12. Positional dimensions and axes helpful in perception. (Excerpted from Olson and Bailystock, 1983.)

The authors also found that instruction which focused on a film representation of complete rotations of objects with accompanying descriptions significantly improved learner's skills in perceiving rotations. They state:

> The critical aspect of instruction was the observation of the transformation that occurs when an object is rotated in space. . . . Appropriate instruction is a powerful alternative to direct experience in the development of a spatial skill. (pp. 180–81)

They go on to state that "a verbal training procedure in which just those critical spatial relations were specified" would not only improve initial performance but also increase the transfer of learning to problems which involve similar representations and operations (p. 181).

Direct training in spatial perception (e.g., comparisons, orientation) should be introduced and formally taught during laboratory components of basic science courses with a focus on cells, organs, etc., and reinforced during the clinical years during rotations which involve patient care: surgery, radiology, etc. Specific functions or tasks required during the preclinical years which involve spatial perceptual skills include sectioning, rotating, and observing demonstrations and slides which require visualizing three-dimensional physical objects. During the clinical years, skills ranging from placing an IV and suturing, to reading and interpreting x-rays and MRI depend heavily upon spatial perceptual skills. Students not only will perform better on exams and lab practicals but also will have developed a learning skill integral to their professional careers.

The importance of spatial perception as a learning skill should not be underestimated. Research has demonstrated that the more developed a student's spatial perceptual skills, the better his or her academic performance in the laboratory practical component of anatomy exams. In this regard, Rochford (1985) found that medical students who failed a series of geometrical (three-dimensional) spatial exercises and/or did more poorly on spatially oriented questions on exams (relative to non-spatially oriented questions) scored significantly lower on lab practicals in anatomy than did those students who scored well in the geometrical spatial exercises.[1] He hypothesized that failure in this area was related to a lack of preparation and training and that remediation of spatial perceptual skills would improve performance.

You should *assess* your own spatial perceptual needs by comparing your performance on spatially oriented exam questions with performance on non-spatial questions. Course coordinators and faculty in anatomy and pathology should monitor students' performances on these two types of questions and inform them of discrepancies. When discrepancies are identified which might indicate spatial perceptual difficulties, you should practice the strategies identified above. If these difficulties persist, you can determine the extent of your problems and seek assistance in practicing the strategies from a learning specialist (see Chapter 5 for screening guidelines).

It would be helpful for all students to be introduced to spatial perceptual exercises early in their medical education during relevant course work (e.g., the first few classes of gross anatomy). A *screening test* consisting of spatial and non-spatial questions could be used to help students *identify weaknesses* so that it isn't mistakenly assumed that only a select few will benefit from such intervention. It should be noted that one study found that those students in the *middle range* in performance of these skills actually benefitted most from extra instruction in these skills (Brinkman, 1966). Once identified, students can work on exercises to strengthen their spatial perceptual abilities independently or in groups. These exercises should focus on developing strategies of: (1) differentiation or discrimination, (2) identification (recognition and labeling), (3) organization or relationship, and (4) orientation.

Learning Through Kinesthetic Sensori-Motor Skills

Observation skills also include the use of tactile skills. In this regard, the AAMC (1978) technical standards for medical education state: "Observation necessitates the functional use of the sense of vision and somatic sensation." These somatic or tactile skills are very important for gathering information from patients through implementation of clinical examination techniques such as palpation, auscultation, percussion, etc. These clinical skills rely on basic fine and gross motor learning skills.

Gardner (1983) identifies bodily-kinesthetic ability as one of six types of intelligence.[2] He states: "Characteristic of such an intelligence is the ability to use one's body in highly differentiated and skilled ways, for expressive as well as goal directed purposes..." (p. 206). The underlying learning skills involve control of fine and gross motor movements and sensations. Bartlett (1958) describes the process as:

> ...the continuing flow from signals occurring outside the performer and interpreted by him to actions carried out; then on to further signals and more action, up to the culminating point of the achievement of the task, or of whatever part of the task is the immediate objective. (p. 14)

Establishing direction for the task, eliciting and interpreting feedback and repetition differentiate motor-kinesthetic skill from simple behavior or action. As Bartlett (1958) says:

> ...we begin to use the term *skill* only when a good many receptor and effector functions are interlinked and related within an order of significant succession which possesses an inherent character of direction and moves towards an issue regarded as its natural terminus. (p. 13)

Gardner (1983) helps us delineate some of the strategies necessary to accomplish this skill. They include:

> ...a well-honed sense of timing, where each bit of a sequence fits into the stream in an exquisitely placed and elegant way; points of repose or shift, where one phase of the behavior is at an end, and some calibration is necessary before the second one comes into play; a sense of direction, a clear goal to which the sequence has been heading, and a point of no return, where further

input of signals no longer produces a result because the final phase of the sequence has already been activated. (p. 208)

From these descriptions we can define three strategies which should be developed and used by medical students to enhance bodily-kinesthetic skills. They are *directedness, utilizing feedback,* and *timing.* Learners should apply these strategies to the development of specific physical exam skills during the learning process and continually use them to ensure maximum performance. Faculty in courses like physical diagnosis and the clinical clerkships should ensure that they are taught. Depending upon the ultimate goal or task, employment of these strategies may or may not involve the use of specific tools or instruments.

Directedness

This strategy involves the clear identification of the precise outcomes which you want to achieve and the potential ways in which they can be achieved. Knowledge required to make these decisions may come from written or oral instructions, from observation of others, and/or from experience.

Goal setting involves having a clear picture of the desired outcomes before you begin. Once you have defined your outcome(s), you need to identify the methods you will use to achieve them. This is the process of establishing and maintaining direction. Bartlett (1958) states: "So far as skilled movements are concerned, this direction has to be regarded as a property which belongs, or comes to belong, objectively to the movements themselves as they are performed" (p. 19). Included are those which indicate you have performed the skill incorrectly.

One technique for improving directedness is *mental rehearsal.* This involves picturing in your mind the steps and outcomes of the action prior to its initiation. Specifically, you must consider the context while systematically envisioning going through each of the movements and anticipating the results. Studies have demonstrated that this type of mental practice is very effective in developing fine motor behavior (Richardson, 1967). Newell (1981) contends that this strategy is probably most effective in the early stages of skill acquisition.

Utilizing Feedback

Performance improves with one's ability to elicit and recognize feedback during the implementation of a physical exam skill. Generally, feedback comes from the action itself or from the environment in relation to the goal of the action. The feedback is used to modify the action by comparing it to a standard or *schema* (Bartlett, 1961) which has been developed from knowledge or from previous experiences. We could conceive of this schema as a set of rules or principles for learning new kinesthetic responses (Marteniuk, 1978). When feedback is received, either the action is modified, the schema is adapted, or the action continues on course. At least four features of the schema play an important role in determining the course of action. Brooks and Stoney (1971) identify three: force, velocity, and displacement. Marteniuk (1978) adds timing. Developing kinesthetic learning skills requires attention to feedback in relation to each of these features. Feedback can be generated visually as well as kinesthetically. Visual feedback is more important in early motor-kinesthetic learning. In this regard, Holding (1981) states:

> ... in most tasks the early stages of skill tend to rely heavily upon visual feedback, with kinaesthetic cues from the joints, tendons, and muscles assuming greater importance as the skill develops to the point where the learner can *do it blindfold.* (p. 6)

Feedback can be used to enhance learning during the action as well as after the action. Accepting feedback during the action requires an openness to the possibility of making errors. In fact, evidence suggests that errors in details of generally appropriate actions may be *helpful* to retention of the specific skill (Williams & Rodney, 1978) and the ability to generalize the skill to other learning situations (Newell & Shapiro, 1976).

Attending to feedback after an action is an extremely important strategy for kinesthetic skill learning. In this connection, it is important to obtain knowledge of results as soon after the action as possible and to ensure that the level of detail is sufficient to modify action the next time around (if necessary). It is important to search for feedback even if one feels confident in the results of an action. What happened and how it happened should be interpreted in light of what was supposed to happen and how it should have happened (Newell, 1981).

Timing

Timing is another important component of bodily-kinesthetic skills. It is the temporal sequence in which signals and responses to signals are ordered. As Bartlett (1958) says:

...it seems as if it is the near future—*anticipation of what is coming next* if a psychological description is required—that plays the principal part in producing that objective smoothness of performance which is the hallmark of a high quality of skill. (p. 15)

Timing is developed through *practice*. Practice is the repetition of an action or behavior (skill) with the intention of improving performance. It is practice that *hones* the skill and improves the timing among component actions. In medical school, practice enables learners to integrate previously learned skills into higher order, more complex skills, rather than simply assume that this integration will take place.

The literature concerning motor skills provides some guidance for effective practice. Newell (1981) found that all of the following characteristics of practice improve performance of a skill: (1) practice immediately after instructions or a demonstration of a skill; (2) increasing the number of trials or repetitions of a skill within a practice session; and (3) extending practice sessions over a longer period of time. He also suggests that, if possible, it is important to practice the *whole* skill rather than separating it into parts and either practicing them separately or sequentially. If, however, the skill is too complex to learn as a whole, then, at least initially, it should be divided into discrete or sequential parts depending upon how they fit together.

The development of bodily-kinesthetic learning skills often includes the use of other learning skills. For example, Gardner (1983) suggests that practice with objects or tools should focus on the integration of fine motor and spatial-perceptual skills. He states:

Particularly during the initial use of an object or a tool, the individual should carefully coordinate the information that he can assimilate through his spatial intelligence, with the capacities that he has elaborated through his bodily intelligence. Confined to spatial intelligence, he may understand a mechanism reasonably well yet have no idea of how actually to manipulate or operate the object in which it is housed; restricted to bodily intelligence, he may be able to execute the appropriate motions, yet fail to appreciate the way in which the apparatus or the procedure works and therefore be stymied should he encounter it in a somewhat different setting, format or situation. (p. 232)

Marked absence of directedness, attention to feedback, or timing, or inability to perform tasks which rely on bodily-kinesthetic skill lead to learning problems in the clinical years. However, it could also indicate a physical disability which requires therapeutic intervention and/or accommodation by the medical school environment (e.g., modified physical examination objectives which require the ability to direct a physician's assistant to palpate). In such instances, the range is narrowed for learning or developing fine and gross motor skills under normal teaching conditions or independently outside of the class or exam room. In these instances, emphasis should be placed on *reasonably* accommodating to individual differences so that technical standards can be met.

Endnotes

1. An example (from Rochford, 1985) of the type of multiple-choice question in anatomy which demands proficient spatial perceptual skill is:

   (c) A transverse section of the midbrain at the level of the superior colliculus will show:

      (1) the substantia nigra
      (2) the oculomotor nucleus
      (3) the red nucleus
      (4) *the trochlear nerve nucleus
      (5) all four statements are correct

   Select the INCORRECT statement from statements 1–4, or choose 5 if all four statements are correct.

   An example of a question which does not demand the use of this skill is:

   (a) Nerve tracts usually classified as commissures include:

      (1) the cingulum
      (2) *the corpus callosum
      (3) ventral spinothalamic
      (4) corticospinal
      (5) none of the above

        (* indicates the correct answer)

2. The other five forms are: linguistic, musical, logical-mathematical, spatial and personal.

Chapter 2

APPLYING KNOWLEDGE
TO GAIN NEW KNOWLEDGE

MEMORIZING

M emorizing means storing encoded (meaningful) information which becomes knowledge. This knowledge can be retrieved for simple recital or, more importantly, for application tasks such as problem solving or communication. Memorization skills are the learning skills which enable you to develop and to continually renew a sound knowledge base which is essential to any application task. I believe that attributing meaning (encoding) is the essential feature of memorizing and is an important prerequisite to *using* knowledge. This feature makes memorizing an *active* learning process and ultimately improves recall and retention.

The term memorizing has negative connotations today. This stems from the view that memorizing has minimal value and is somehow detached from the thinking process. This perception that memory and thinking are separate and *unequal* is not new. J. P. Guilford (1962), a noted author and scholar in the area of creative thinking, observed this same phenomenon some 30 years ago:

> Many people, including some teachers, have for some reason disparaged memory and memory abilities. Some of them, who emphasize the importance of thinking, seem wrongly to believe that good thinking and good memory are incompatible qualities, perhaps even negatively correlated. Actually, good memory contributes to good thinking. (p. 388)

Memorization is often perceived as passive or *rote* and considered an end in and of itself (viz., recital) rather than as a means to *higher order*, application learning. This *devaluation* often is supported by the curriculum. Rarely is material selected for inclusion in a course by a teacher, and ultimately for memorization by the learner, because it is (or will be) useful in problem solving or communication. Typically course coordinators select material to *cover a topic* and collectively, though unintentionally, *overburden* students with too much information to memorize. Much of the material is of questionable utility. It is imperative that medical students be trained in techniques of effective memorizing and that this training be complemented by a parallel movement to ensure that only information ultimately relevant to application tasks will be required.

Barrows (1985) and many other problem-solving theorists fail to recognize the active nature of effective memorizing. He refers to "the passive memorization of knowledge from lectures and readings" (p. 2) and describes memorizing as a method of learning in which the student is not actively involved in the learning process. His view of memorizing highlights not only the failure of medical educators to define and teach effective memorizing skills but also to fully understand the component parts of problem solving.

Barrows (1985) suggests that memorization is improved by tying the focal content to cues from the clinical context (viz., problem-based learning). These cues would be embedded in a specific case. It is precisely this process of generating external associative cues, however, that inhibits generalization of knowledge. It is more important to establish *internal* meaning first.

Consider the process of remembering the origins, products and function of B and T lymphocytes in a case which involves a patient with HIV. The overriding focus is likely to be on the devastation of the immune system as opposed to its protective properties. By virtue of the specific case, the details emphasized, and associative cues developed, are different than they would be in another case, say, for example, the acceptance/rejection of a transplanted organ. By not learning about the general, inherent properties and characteristics of B & T lymphocytes, we are less likely to transfer the knowledge especially when cases are very different.

Although associating information to be learned with specific contextual cues (e.g., clinical) is one method of attributing meaning, it is less effective than initially finding meaning inherent in the information. First, as our example suggests, memorized information tied to cues from a specific clinical context may inhibit later generalizability of the knowledge to other clinical problems and contexts because these or similar cues are not present. That is, the greater the difference between external cues employed during memorization and those present at retrieval, the less the chance of retrieval. In one sense, Barrows (1985) is correct when he states that: "Learning in a clinical context causes the information that is being acquired to be organized or structured in the mind in ways that are useful to clinical tasks" (p. 4). It may, however, be useful to only a very prescribed set of clinical tasks.

Information memorized using external cues also is less well understood in terms of rules and principles which govern its use. In this regard, failure to find meaning in the structure of knowledge itself will likely inhibit creative modification of that knowledge. In the example above, learning about the inherent properties and characteristics of B and T lymphocytes by comparing, contrasting, and other forms of establishing internal meaning, will likely ensure that this information can be applied to dissimilar and perhaps novel contexts, retrieved and later used in the clinical context in creative ways.

In medical school the demands for remembering information have increased dramatically. This is coupled with the fact that most medical students have no formal training in memorizing and have no strategies for handling the increased volume. Students rely upon repetition, cramming and other methods of rote learning which were generally sufficient when needed to do well on *recognition* oriented tests (e.g., multiple choice) in high school or college. These rote learning strategies, however, fail to help retrieve basic science knowledge for application to problem-solving tasks (Boshuizen & Schmidt, 1990). The reason is that rote memory may suffice for recognition (e.g., choosing the correct alternative to a multiple-choice question) but active memory is required for *recall* which is necessary for problem solving.

As Boshuizen and Schmidt (1990) state:

> ...although people may know a certain thing, there is no guarantee that this knowledge will always be accessed—neither when the student is asked for it directly, nor when indirect questions are posed, nor *when the student is confronted with problems in which that knowledge is supposed to be applied.* Evocation of specific knowledge depends on the availability of context cues associated with that knowledge (Tulving & Thompson, 1971) and on the flexibility and accessibility of the larger knowledge structures in which it is embedded. Failure to apply relevant knowledge may result in an imprecise or even completely wrong diagnosis. (p. 221)

It is clear that *both* context cues and structural characteristics of knowledge play important roles in retrieving knowledge and ultimately defining the effectiveness of memorization. Students will benefit from developing appropriate strategies related to both of these areas for memorizing greater volume with the intent of applying knowledge.

Medical school requires that learners invest new energy in the memorization process. Often this entails learning new strategies to enhance effectiveness. Consider the analogy of learning to drive a car (Ornstein et al., 1988):

> In the early stages of learning, the coordination of the clutch, accelerator, and brake pedals is not particularly smooth. . . . Later the various operations are integrated somewhat, and subjectively it appears as if driving is a less effortful task. . . . However, even when driving seems to require little conscious attention, changes in the road or traffic conditions may again require the investment of most of the driver's resources in the demands of driving the car. (pp. 37–38)

Changes in the road and traffic conditions in the memorization lane of medical school may be likened to entering the Los Angeles freeway during rush hour after a leisurely drive on a country road in college.

The first strategy in memorizing is deciding what to memorize. Medical students do not have the time to memorize everything they hear in class or at rounds, or that they read in journals, books, or class handouts. They do not have time to memorize everything they are required to remember. For many students this is a problem of major proportions. They don't or can't decide *what to memorize.* In response to the work load, students may try to memorize everything, or simply read and not try to *actively* memorize anything. Either response may be accompanied by anxiety or depression.

This strategy involves selecting information to be remembered which you think is important. Two criteria should be used in making this selection; utility and probability. First, assess the *utility* of the material. Will it be useful to me on the test? To solve problems? As a physician? Ultimately, memorizing should be viewed as an active process of incorporating information which is of interest for the purpose of using it (e.g., problem solving) at a later date (cf., Bruner, 1961). However, often it is important to pay attention to short-term goals such as passing an exam.

To assess utility, develop your own rating system (e.g., one to ten) which can be used regularly with *all* material in each course. Your assessment should be based upon your own perceptions as well as information from other sources including professors (viz., emphasis in class, handouts, previous tests), advisors, other students in the class, students from the previous classes, and tutors. It is necessary to develop and prioritize a list of resources and informants necessary to help you make your decisions about utility in each course. Utility of new information is an important criterion for defining importance during *active* memorization.

The second criterion for assessing importance is the probability that the information can be adequately learned in the time available. As you become more familiar with the process of memorizing described below, you will understand the importance of blocking out sufficient time for each memorization task. You also will become more accurate in estimating probability of accomplishment in the alloted time and how this will affect your ability to manage time. Once again, develop a rating system which will help you to quantify the probability of accomplishing a memorization strategy in the amount of available time. The strategy of assigning a probability score ultimately will help you prospectively schedule memorization tasks.

Once you have decided what to memorize, you are ready for the next step in memorizing: focusing your attention on the material at hand. First, in order to devote full attention to the material at hand, it is important that your physical environment be conducive to the task. This means an environment that is free of all distractions (visual, auditory, and other sensory stimuli). It would include, for example, proper lighting, absence of loud noise or music, and fulfillment of basic needs (such as nourishment, sleep, etc.).

Once these contextual determinants of attention have been addressed, it is important to focus on your relationship with the material itself. This involves finding meaning in the material. Making memorizing an active process by attributing meaning to the material increases your attention (Cermack, 1975). Memorizing must be viewed as a creative and productive mental process. With reference to the learner who is memorizing, Crutchfield (1969) states:

> He must render the fact relevant and meaningful, and he must do this through a process of directed mental activity which has as its end the complete ingesting, metabolizing, and incorporating of the fact in such a way that it becomes widely "distributed" throughout the diverse reaches of his conceptual system. (p. 56)

The importance of meaning to memory has been demonstrated in experimental research. These studies have found that conceptual processing (viz., finding meaning) during studying is integral to effective recall and recognition. Snodgrass and Hirshman (1994) conclude from their review of the literature, "success on explicit tests such as recognition and recall depends on conceptual processing at study—on having stored the meaning of the studied item" (p. 151).

The first step in finding meaning in new information is to let your mind search *known* information for associations. Ultimately, how well one is able to integrate new information with, and differentiate new information from, *old* knowledge will determine how well one remembers or retains the new information. Consider the task of remembering the specifics of: (1) Wernicke's aphasia: a lesion in the planum temporale, a common manifestation of dementia, and absence of understanding of spoken words; and (2) Broca's aphasia: right hemiplegia: a lesion centered in the left inferior frontal gyrus resulting in absence of, or severely limited, speech and writing ability. Remembering these specifics is enhanced by previous basic knowledge that in the left hemisphere, Wernicke's area provides more detailed commands, error signals, and correction signals to Broca's area for the production of language via the *arcuate fasciculus.*

The search for associations focuses on knowledge which we have previously organized to facilitate recall. In this connection, Miller (1956) suggests that we can remember a list of familiar words more effectively than we can remember a list of nonsense words. This would suggest that the more we can organize new information based upon previous knowledge, the more likely we will be to remember it. In addition, the larger we can *chunk* new information, the less we have to create new units of association, and once again, the more we will remember. In this connection, Miller (1956) states: "Since the memory span is a fixed number of chunks, we can increase the number of bits of information that it contains simply by building larger and larger chunks, each chunk containing more information than before" (p. 93). In the example of aphasia cited above, we are expanding the chunk of our knowledge of the parts of the brain responsible for language. To effectively remember this information, we must *file* it in this larger *folder.*

The next strategy is to create general categories, and use principles of organization, to make sense of the new information. As in focused reading, the first step is to translate new information into *your own words.* Rewrite or restate it without rereading it and in such a way as the meaning is perfectly clear. The next step is to use principles such as function, commonalities, differences, causal relationships, outcomes, etc., to group the details. In the above example we could say that the two types of aphasia (commonality) represent damage to two parts of the brain required for two separate, but interrelated language functions (difference): production (Broca's) and understanding (Wernicke's). Although both types inhibit communication function, they do so for very different reasons (causal relations) and the behavioral manifestations (outcomes) are quite different.

This method of simplifying representation of detailed material by applying general or fundamental underlying principles helps to create a pathway for memory which begins with recall of the general and then allows for association of the details. For example, when we use a principle like commonality (e.g., both effect language functions) we may initially recall some (production and understanding are differentiated) but not all of the characteristics. However, remembering this major characteristic may *trigger* the *second order* characteristic of the relationship to dementia. Bruner (1960) goes on to say:

> . . . knowledge one has acquired without sufficient structure to tie it together is knowledge that is likely to be forgotten. An unconnected set of facts has a pitiably short half-life in memory. Organizing facts in terms of principles and ideas from which they may be inferred is the only way of reducing the quick rate of loss of human memory. (pp. 31–32)

Organizing new material in meaningful ways improves both storage and retrieval, the two stages of remembering. Storage is, as the word suggests, the process of placing the material in memory. It is during storage that organizing is a premier learning strategy. The second aspect is retrieval, which may include either recall or recognition. Recognition involves remembering with the aid of a sensory cue (e.g., one of four alternatives to a multiple-choice question) to *boost* the memory process. Recall, on the other hand, involves remembering spontaneously without cues or by *willing* it to happen.

Organizing information up front in the memorization process facilitates storage and enhances retrieval by enabling later recall to more closely approximate the process of recognition. As we know, under most circumstances, recognition is easier than recall. Research has determined that retention as measured through recognition is as much as three times higher than retention measured through recall (Adams, 1967). This finding does not hold true when the number of false alternatives in a recognition test is too high (e.g., a matching question involving 15 alternatives).

Another factor, which greatly influences the superiority of recognition over recall, is the discriminability of the alternatives. If there are alternatives which are difficult to distinguish among, then retention will be as low or lower than in recall because of the distraction factor. Organizational aids serve as intermediary cues to aid recall in much the same way that sensory cues act to boost recognition.

Knowledge (memorized information) that is organized meaningfully will also improve the *applicability* of what is retrieved. Guilford (1962) states:

> It is the way in which storage is achieved and organized that makes the difference between the graduate who is sometimes described as "merely a walking encyclopedia" and the graduate who has a usable and fruitful fund of information. Memory abilities thus make their indirect but important contribution to creative performance. (p. 388)

How well, and in what form, you organize information during storage will determine how well you can retrieve that information. The key is to enhance the *conditions* of recognition even under circumstances of recall. Bruner (1961) states that:

> We may infer this from the fact that recognition (i.e., recall with the aid of maximum prompts) is so extraordinarily good in human beings—particularly in comparison with spontaneous recall where, so to speak, we must get out stored information without external aids or prompts. The key to retrieval is organization or, in even simpler terms, knowing where to find information and how to get there. (p. 31)

Organizational cues should act as *bridges* between the stored or retained information and the context in which the information will be used. Consider the information on protective immunization provided in Figure 13.

Disease	Causative Agent	Type of Vaccine	Duration of Protection
Measles	Virus	Live	Long-lasting
Tetanus	Bacterium	Toxoid	Long-lasting
Tularemia	Bacterium	Killed	Short-lived
Mumps	Virus	Live	Long-lasting
Typhoid Fever	Bacterium	Killed	Short-lived

Figure 13. Protective immunization. (Excerpted from Mellinkoff, 1973.)

The first step in organizing this information is to *chunk* it by major meaning groups; similarities in causative agent (virus vs. bacterium), type of vaccine (live vs. killed vs. other) *or* duration of protection (long-lasting vs. short-lived) depending on the nature of expected retrieval. For example, if the intended context of retrieval is an exam in an immunology course, then perhaps *causative* agent is the most important initial organizational cue. On the other hand, if the intended context of retrieval is clinical practice, then the most important cue might be *duration of protection.*

Bruner (1961) gives a simple demonstration of the importance of organizers to storage and recall. It also illustrates the importance of allowing the learner to define his/her own organizers. In his study, children were presented pairs of words. One group was given no direction other than they would be asked to repeat them later. The second group was told to remember them by making up a word that will tie the two words together. Children in the second group recalled second words in the pair 95 percent of the time compared to 50 percent in the first group. A third group which was given the organizing words developed by the second group fared in between, strongly suggesting the importance of *personal* mediating cues.

In the case of memorizing the items in the protective immunization table, you might first group the diseases by causative agent, then by duration of protection, and finally consider your own or your family's history of immunizations in relation to these organizational cues. Have you been immunized for tetanus, measles, or mumps? How long does it last?

In this sense the process of memorization may be likened to the process of problem solving. Once the data is gathered, we search for the best way to organize it for either hypothesis formulation as in problem solving, or for recall, as in memorizing. Together with selecting and assigning probability, organizing and assigning personal meaning makes memorizing an extremely active learner-centered process.

Grouping information is an essential feature of developing meaningful organizers. There are many ways in which this can be accomplished. One is to use descriptors identified earlier in the discussion of spatial perception. For example, we can group data by similarities and/or differences of function (e.g., direction, speed) or of structure (e.g., shape, size, level of generality/specificity, proximity).

We know that grouping is a developmentally advanced form of thinking, thus making it particularly relevant to adult learning. In this regard, there is evidence that grouping or organizing into meaning units is common among adults and not among children when faced with undirected tasks of memorizing material (Naus & Orenstein, 1983). There is also evidence of a positive association between degree of organization and successful recall (Naus & Orenstein, 1983). These and other research findings would strongly support the importance of developing and practicing effective organizational behaviors (viz., grouping) as an important strategy for memorizing.

The strategy of grouping should be linked with preferred learning style (see Chapter 4 on learning differences) to enhance its effectiveness. For example, grouping by either part-whole or means-ends relationships can be particularly effective for *visual* learners. During study, this can be accomplished using visual imagery (viz., imagination) or by actually drawing figural relations on paper. With respect to the former, Tulving (1983) cites research in which subjects, who were instructed to use visual imagery to encode material to be remembered, demonstrated greater retention than those who were given no such instructions.

To enhance memory for the visual learner, figural representations with component parts presented in relation to each other, and in relation to the whole, also can be drawn using lines, shapes and forms. These figures or diagrams have been called *mind maps* (Gross, 1991). Generally, *mind maps* begin with the main topic in the center and work their way out with details and sub-details. However, you can develop your own rules for creating these maps, deriving personal meaning through such features as direction, color, space, proximity, etc. In fact, research would suggest that personally *coded* maps are most effective for memorizing. Consider the following (mini) mind map (Figure 14) constructed from information in a physiology handout.

Using mnemonics is a special case of recoding input material which helps to improve memory (Miller, 1956). A mnemonic is an example of an organizer which combines internal meaning with extrinsic cues. Material is first organized by recoding or chunking information into smaller units based on intrinsic meaning. Finally, it is tied to an external structure along with rules for decoding and then stored. For purposes of retrieval, the organization process is reversed. With use, decreasing numbers of external cues are necessary for retrieval.

The organizing principle of a mnemonic is found in the external cues. "Mnemonics seek to impose order on material that you want to remember rather than seeking order within the material itself" (Cermack, 1975, p. 97). Bellezza (1981) defines a mnemonic as:

> . . . a strategy for organizing and/or encoding information with the sole purpose of making it more memorable. . . . These cognitive cuing structures are typically made up of either visual images or of words in the form of sentences or rhymes. Their general purpose is to act as mediators between the

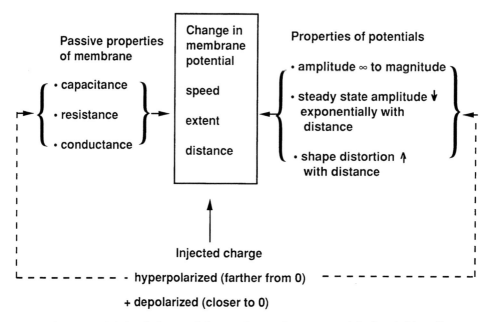

Figure 14. (Mini) mind-map of changes in membrane potential of excitable cells.

signal to the learner to recall and the information to be remembered. . . . The cuing structure used to remember a set of information is often not conceptually related to the information it cues. (p. 252)

The most common mnemonics used in the study of medicine are what Bellezza (1981) calls *single-use* mnemonics. In this case, a new and distinct set of associative cues is created for each set of material to be remembered. Typically the cues are first letters in the words or sets of words to be remembered. These cues are arranged to form a new word or sentence which may have little or nothing to do with the meaning of the words to be remembered. The fabricated word or sentence (external cue) serves as a trigger for the associated words and their meanings (internal meaning). As Bellezza (1981) states: "When trying to recall this information the mnemonic is recalled first along with the rules for decoding it. It then acts as a set of retrieval cues extrinsic to the information that is desired" (p. 257).

Several predefined mnemonics are available in the medical literature and commonly used to aid memory. CAGE is a common word mnemonic in clinical medicine where each letter serves as a cue for components of an alcohol abuse screening instrument:

CAGE

In the past three months:

- Have you felt the need to Cut down on your drinking?
- Has anyone Annoyed you or gotten on your nerves by telling you to cut down on your drinking?
- Have you ever felt Guilty or bad about how much you drink?
- Have you woken with the need for an Eye-opener?

Another word mnemonic commonly used in clinical medicine is the Apgar instrument used to assess newborns:

APGAR

- How is the neonate's Appearance and color?
- What is her/his Pulse?
- Is there a Grimace (reflex, irritability)?
- How is Activity?
- How is Respiratory effort?

The first words in a sentence also can serve as external cues in a mnemonic. Consider the sentence: "Good Students Give Loving Care." The first letter in each word represents epidermis layers from base to surface: stratum Germinativum, stratum Spinosum, stratum Granulosum, stratum Lucidum, stratum Conium (Bhushan et al., 1993). A sample of other word and sentence mnemonics defined by Bhushan et al. (1993) can be found in Figure 15.

Although many predefined mnemonics are available, you should realize that defining *your own* mnemonics will gain you the most mileage in terms of memory. As Bruner's (1961) research on personal cues as mediators would suggest, the more personal meaning this created word or sentence has, the easier it will be to use the mnemonic later. This is an important point to remember when using mnemonics. It is better to create your own *meaningful* mnemonic than it is to adopt one that already exists.

One of the oldest documented types of mnemonic which uses space as the organizing feature is the *method of loci*. This technique which is generally referred to as a *receptacle* mnemonic is underutilized by learners in medicine. It dates back to early Roman times and was used to improve rhetoric (Yates, 1966). Bellezza (1981) describes a lecturer's use of the *method of loci* in this way:

CONCEPT	DESCRIPTION	MNEMONIC ---------------------------------- WORD
Leukocyte	Types: granulocytes (basophils, eosinophils, neutrophils) and mononuclear cells (lymphocytes, monocytes). Responsible for defense against infections. Normally 4,000-10,000 per microliter.	Leuko = white. Think of BEN-GRAy: Basophils, Eosinophils, and Neutrophils are GRAnulocytes.
Cornea	1. S tratified epithelium 2. B owman's membrane 3. S troma 4. D escemet's membrane 5. S imple endothelium; continuous with sclera (at limbus)	The cornea SuBSiDeS into the sclera.
Brunner's glands	Secrete alkaline mucus. Located in submucosa of duodenum (the only GI submucosal gland).	BAGS: B runner's A lkaline G lands, S ubmucosal
Rotator cuff muscles	Shoulder muscles that form the rotator cuff: S upraspinatus, I nfraspinatus, t eres minor, S ubscapularis.	SItS (small t is for teres minor).
		SENTENCE
Ureters: course	Ureters pass UNDER uterine artery and UNDER ductus deferens.	Water (uterers) UNDER the bridge (artery).
Kubler-Ross dying stages	Denial, Anger, Bargaining, Grieving, Acceptance.	Death Arrives Bringing Grave Adjustments

Figure 15. Word and sentence mnemonics. (Excerpted from Bhushan et al., 1993.)

First, a large number of places in some public building were memorized in a strict serial order, such that each locus could be clearly visualized from memory. Then, after a speech was prepared, its content was reduced to a series of visual images, where each image represented an important word or idea in a speech. Each of these images was then "placed" or associated with the corresponding locus in the same ordinal position as the image. During his speech the orator would mentally visualize each locus in turn and, using it as a cue, recall the associated mental image. The mental image acted as a prompt for the next part of the speech. (p. 254)

This technique has been used with dramatic results by professional memorizers, or *mnemonists*. Take, for example, Sherashevsky (S.), the Russian mnemonist described by A.R. Luria, the eminent Russian physician and psychologist. Luria (1987) described S. as having a "virtual unlimited memory." When presented with series of words, letters, or numbers, he could reproduce them forwards, backwards or begin and end at any place in between. Luria (1987) states:

> An increase in the length of a series led to no noticeable increase in difficulty for S., and I simply had to admit that the capacity of his memory *had no distinct limits;* that I had been unable to perform what one would think was the simplest task a psychologist can do: measure the capacity of an individual's memory. (p. 11)

Not only could S. remember lists of thirty, fifty or seventy words or numbers, he could recall them fifteen or sixteen years later. During memorization he would associate graphic images with each word or number to be recalled. When there were long lists he would incorporate a temporal or graphic sequence of images on which to *hang* the sequential information to be learned. As Luria (1987) states: "He would distribute them along some [familiar] roadway or street he visualized in his mind," (p. 32) and "he would simply begin his walk, either from the beginning or from the end of the street, find the image of the object I had named, and take a look at whatever happened to be situated on either side of it" (p. 33).

This technique is particularly well suited for the student with strong *visual learning* capacity. Use the following exercise to determine the usefulness of this mnemonic technique in memorizing the features of the digestive tube presented in Figure 16.

Exercise

Picture a room in your apartment or house. In your mind, walk through the room in a clockwise direction choosing eighteen key objects. Study the following diagram of the digestive tube. Begin at the lymphoid nodule and proceed clockwise, associating each feature of the tube with an object in the room. Make sure that you understand each feature in relation to each other, and the entire tube.

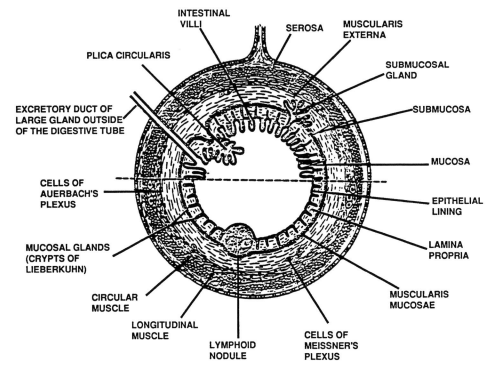

Figure 16. The digestive tube.

Some types of information to be remembered are more conducive to being organized in receptacle mnemonics than others. Sequences of information, chains of causally related material, and related parts of a whole, like the example above, are most compatible with this technique. It is also important to note that this technique takes practice; the loci must be solidly entrenched in memory and practiced often. Material which has been organized (viz., is meaningful) and only needs to be boosted for short periods of time (e.g., in preparation for a presentation, test or quiz) could be reinforced using the method of loci technique. Each student who uses this technique should examine his/her own limits to recycling loci.

An efficiency feature of this technique is that the receptacles (e.g., room, house, street) can be recycled for future use. However, some research has shown that new images associated with the loci may tend to interfere with the old ones (Bellezza, 1981). Although the research findings are inconclusive, this could place restrictions on what material should be memorized with this technique. Suffice to say that you should not use the same receptacle to remember sets of similar information for the same exam.

It is also important to remember that if mnemonics are to be used, they should be used with information which already has been organized or structured into meaning units. The underlying principle of a mnemonic is to provide cues which will aid recall. If the material recalled has no internal meaning, then it is *practically* useless. Using mnemonics to enhance memory does not enhance understanding, and jumping too quickly to implement a mnemonic without first finding meaning in the material will be detrimental to learning and to the practice of medicine.

There is research evidence which suggests that as material originally memorized using a mnemonic is used more often (viz., material which is more important), *mediating mnemonics* are no longer needed for recall and more direct links in meaning are strengthened to enhance memory (Belleza, 1981). In effect, intrinsic meaning supplants extrinsic cues as one becomes more experienced. This would argue effectively for greater use of mnemonics and may silence critics who question the retention and level of understanding involved in this type of learning. One might, in fact, argue that with all of the information medical students are expected to memorize, that information which is of questionable use in later learning or practice, or which will be *built upon,* could most efficiently be stored in a *holding pattern* in mnemonic memory. As future experience and need dictates (viz., that information which is used most often), the most important knowledge will become more solidly entrenched and recalled using intrinsic meaning cues.

Another important strategy for organizing information to be remembered is to consider, even predict, how the information will or could ultimately be used (in problem solving, communication, etc.). Each time you are presented with information to be remembered, think about the potential applications to learning and practice. *Challenge* yourself to use the information in multiple forms. This flexibility of knowledge should aid recall.

This is quite different than being told how to use the information; a procedure often followed in problem-based learning (Barrows, 1985). Even if you are instructed to generalize, it is not the same as discovering that it can be done yourself. The latter can lead to a kind of academic *myopia* or *parochialism* in learning which is difficult to undo. Learners may only associate knowledge with the narrow range of cues with which they are presented and fail to understand the generalizable quality of the retained information. This can lead to what Bruner (1961) calls "over-specialization of information processing that may lead to such a high degree of specific organization that information is lost for general use" (p. 26). In other words, students who are *spoon-fed* associations and applications of knowledge to specific cases (or types of cases) often fail to generalize this knowledge to other cases (or types).

All of the strategies for remembering considered thus far primarily relate to how you organize the content to be remembered. Although organizing material is a crucial step in memorization, there is also a *process* of memorizing which should be followed.

The first strategy in the process of memorization is *rehearsal.* Rehearsal must include more than *rote* imitation. It should be viewed as an extension of organizing the material with the added goal of developing mental associations (Naus & Ornstein, 1983). In this sense it includes some of the features of developing a mnemonic. One can assume that active rehearsal also enhances attention and helps to maintain the learner's focus.

A great deal of memory research has been done in the area of rehearsal and it is evident that it is an important step in ensuring storage and later recall. Naus and Ornstein (1983) report that differences in rehearsal activity influence how easily a person can retrieve the material from long-term memory. They also found that the *more organized* and structured the material to be remembered (viz., more meaningful), the *less rehearsal* was required, because rehearsal also involves developing associations. This view of rehearsal is more complex than perceived by some authors (cf., Flavell, 1977).

Rehearsal often works best when it takes the form of writing. Written rehearsal facilitates the development of mental associations by reinforcing organizational cues and utilizing other sensory modalities (viz., fine motor and visual). By doing so, it engages the learner's attention and, in many instances (especially during the preclinical years), represents the medium in which retrieval is required (i.e., written exams).

First, active rehearsal should be used to incorporate material into short-term memory once it has been organized. A helpful formula for rehearsal is offered by Willey and Jarecky (1976) who have applied the concept to medical education. The authors describe four *cycles* for rehearsal associated with committing information to short- and long-term memory. The following is a summarized and amended version of their helpful formula.

First, information must be organized using the strategies described above. Once you have accomplished this, analyze it until you are comfortable that you can recreate it. Cover the organized material and attempt to recreate it in written form. Next, *compare* your creation to the original, *highlighting* errors with a different color pen or pencil. This is an important step in that it helps you to focus on the material that you don't know rather than the material you know. Because of our natural tendencies as learners to seek gratification, we often divert our attention while learning to material we already know rather than to material we don't know and must learn. Even the act of highlighting our mistakes tends to focus our rehearsal efforts on that which we don't know instead of being diverted to that which we know. Willey and Jarecky (1976) suggest that we then *throw* the corrected recreation away as a sign that it has been entered in short-term memory. It may be better, however, to keep the corrected version so that highlighted mistakes can be compared to mistakes committed in the long-term memory rehearsal process described below.

The next step is to incorporate the material into your long-term memory. Within a twelve- to twenty-four hour period, you should *rehearse again*, with only the cues that might be expected for retrieval or actual use (e.g., practice test question, title of a chart, table or figure). You should then compare this third version with your previously corrected version, again comparing and highlighting errors. Finally, rehearsal should be used during a review within a few days of expected retrieval to make sure that previously highlighted errors are corrected in memory and that all details are stored properly and available in the near future. During this *dress rehearsal,* only those cues expected during retrieval should be provided as a stimulus to aid recall.

All of the process strategies mentioned thus far have to do with *studying* the material in preparation for eventual use. Another set of process strategies for aiding memory focuses on the act of retrieval (Flavell, 1977). *Memory facilitators* are principles of remembering which should be followed during retrieval. The first is to be *persistent* during retrieval. In this regard, Flavell (1977) insists you "not . . . give up your memory search immediately just because the sought-for item does not come to mind immediately" (p. 204). The strategy is to return *regularly* to test questions you *feel* you know but cannot answer, searching generally in the area of your memory (i.e., knowledge of the topic) which it *could* be found. The strategy of returning regularly to unanswered questions also allows new insights gained from reading and answering subsequent questions to possibly be used.

Another memory facilitator involves using the sensory stimuli of the learning context as an associative cue. For example, cues from the environment, or your transactions with the environment, during learning will help invoke recall. Picturing in your mind the lecturer, the classroom, the time, the page in your notebook or the drawing that you created and studied are all examples of this type of secondary stimuli. This is much like using the *method of loci* except that the loci are retrospectively recalled from the actual learning context. Like mnemonic devices, these recollected contextual characteristics which are transformed into graphic images *ground* your memory, spatially and temporally, and have very little directly to do with the meaning of the material. The importance of setting is grounded in the *functionalist* perspective of memory in psychology as popularized by William James at the turn of the century, who argued that "the setting of the to-be-recalled event or experience is an important part of remembering, for it is the setting that makes one recognize the thought as a recollection" (Dixon & Hertzog, 1988, p. 296).

This memory facilitator most certainly can be strengthened by increasing and broadening attention skills employed during the *learning event.* Practice this strategy by taking a couple of minutes during your next lecture to attend to contextual characteristics. When does the lecture begin? When does it end? What are you wearing? What preceded and followed the lecture? What characterized the lecturer? What did she/he look like? Where were you sitting? Who was beside you? Anything unusual about the setting? Later in the day, try to recall the setting characteristics as associative cues for the material presented. Remember that ultimately associative cues will be most helpful when they are tied to material *which has intrinsic meaning.*

Finally, we should consider the importance of medical informatics as a strategy for increasing memory. As stated in the beginning of this chapter there is a paradigm shift in medical education from a focus on learning content to a focus on the process of learning how to use content. This reflects a recognition of the increasing complexity of medicine and medical care and the need to develop new information management strategies to supplement human memory. There is an understanding that the volume of medical content has expanded well beyond the capacity of *old* ways of handling it (e.g., storing it in memory or finding an answer in one of a few medical books). Blois (1984) states:

> Medical educators are increasingly frustrated by the impossibility of communicating this mass of knowledge to the next generation of physicians. And absorbing this knowledge in the near absence of unifying or organizing principles taxes each new generation of medical students ever more severely. (p. xi)

Computers present an effective and efficient aid to memory for purposes of managing information. In order to use computers effectively, medical students must learn to use computer hardware and software to store (encode), manipulate (apply), and access (retrieve) data. These processes *mirror* human learning processes. Specific information management tasks include literature and data base searches, diagnostic consultation, patient chart preparation, and access and report generation. Related learning strategies include word processing, developing and maintaining data bases, networking, statistical analyses, and using computer simulation to develop and refine problem-solving ability. Development of these strategies will: (1) facilitate formal medical education (viz., medical school and residency), (2) contribute to, and enhance, independent lifelong learning, and (3) ultimately improve patient care.

It is beyond the scope of this book to help the learner develop proficiency in each of these learning strategies which involve background and skills in other disciplines. Each is complex, and medical students present with highly variable experience and needs in each area. Suffice to say that the more competent you become in each strategy, the brighter your future in managing the ever-growing plethora of medical information.

One learning strategy which is particularly relevant to the enhancement of memory capacity for clinical purposes is the computerized diagnostic consultation. With the current capability of many clinical data bases in hospitals, clinics, and health centers, the medical student or physician can answer questions using information generated from the experiences of many physicians over a long period of time. Consultation of the past tended to be *hit or miss* and, most often, was based upon the limited experience of one clinician. Now, one need only know how to enter a data base and how to utilize the appropriate commands (ask the appropriate questions). Even utilizing the appropriate commands is becoming an easier task with the development of *natural language* programs. Blois (1984) states that this type of interactive program "makes it possible to make inquiries of a data base by means of questions expressed in natural language, and avoids the need for a user to learn a special query or procedural language or, alternatively, of employing a programmer as an intermediary" (p. 190). He cites the example question which can elicit an intelligent response from a data base in his melanoma clinic: "How many patients with level-2 melanoma have died?" (p. 239).

Of course, utilizing the correct command presumes knowing the right question to ask. In this sense, the informatics strategies are truly application strategies. Without the accompaniment of other memorization strategies, previously described, such as organizing meaningful information, informatics is of little use. It is also important to remember that medical consultation of this sort should be subject to the same scrutiny and clinical judgment as consultation of the past and is not a replacement for thinking.

It is clear that the development of information management skills should be initiated, accomplished, evaluated, and reinforced within the context of the medical school curriculum. As with all of the learning strategies described in this chapter, it is important that faculty and students work together in their development and implementation. It is as inappropriate to expect students to gain proficiency in these lifelong learning strategies on their own as it would be to expect them to learn biochemistry on their own.

Using the strategies described in this section will improve your memory if other factors are controlled. These factors include your: (1) attitude toward, and interest in, the topic; (2) motivation to learn; (3) emotional state (e.g., anxious, depressed); and (4) physical condition of you (e.g., fatigued, hungry) and of your environment (noisy, hot). Careful attention should be paid to each of these personal and environmental factors which can affect ability to store and retrieve information.

PROBLEM-SOLVING SKILLS

Problem solving has received a great deal of attention recently in medical education. So much so that entire curricula are now devoted to problem-based learning (Barrows, 1985). These curricular innovations, which center learning around medical problems, are noble undertakings and underscore the need to emphasize this learning skill from the beginning of medical school. However, most of the curriculum development activity, as described in the medical education literature, has focused on the *process of implementing curricular* innovations and neglected to precisely define the learning strategies necessary to solve medical problems. This unfortunate oversight may result in the adoption of curricula which do not effectively teach problem-solving skills, and also ignore the development of a sound knowledge base from which to solve problems. With respect to the latter, research in the field of problem solving has demonstrated the importance of knowledge to assess the validity of inferences and assertions. Nickerson (1986) states: "Clearly a knowledge-based ability, is essential to effective reasoning in any but the most abstract sense" (p. 359).

Effective medical problem solving is characterized by the ability to generalize or transfer the use of knowledge from one patient-environment context to another. If problem-based learning curricula are to be successful, they must be structured in such a way as to emphasize novelty in analyses of situations, use of techniques, etc. The study problems should be chosen to: (1) exemplify the uniqueness of the situation; (2) contrast totally different uses of the same methods and techniques depending on the characteristics of the patient-environment context; and (3) reflect very different solutions to apparently similar problems. As Vinacke (1952) states, students must learn that:

> It is not a matter of the mechanical application of rules or principles—not just the blind application of operations which have worked before. The solution grows out of an understanding of the specific requirements of the immediate problem. (p. 177)

Problem solving, like reading, memorizing and communicating with others, is a learning skill. It is a Level II skill which means that it involves the integration and use of other learning skills including memorization, perception, etc. It is actually a series of cognitive strategies which, when employed in combination with other learning skills (e.g., communication, physical exam), allows you to learn more about the patient's problem by applying knowledge to gain new knowledge. What you should be learning in problem-based curricula is how to approach each unique clinical problem by analyzing its dynamic, structural and content features. What you should *not* be learning is how to apply specific basic science knowledge to a clinical problem. The latter is an example of *rote* learning and will only stifle the development of effective problem-solving skills. As Vinacke (1952) states:

> Instead of struggling to cope with the situation in a habitual, mechanical, "blind" manner, the individual can construct, or reconstruct, or reorganize

features of the situation in accordance with the inner relations of the problem as a whole. Problem solving, in this way, is conceived to be a dynamic, fluid process. . . . That is, relationships, principles, attitudes, methods, etc., are more significant than specific content, or specific operations, or specific rules. (pp. 177–8)

Barrows (1985) helps us understand the relationship between clinical problem solving and hypothetical-deductive thinking. He uses terms like hypothesize, analyze, synthesize, etc., to describe the problem-solving process. In this section I will define the strategies necessary to learn how to problem solve and the relationship between problem solving and other learning skills. Specific guidelines for practicing problem solving which are helpful for learners and teachers will be presented.

Problem solving involves a series of discrete operational strategies which, when mastered, will enable the learner to most effectively undertake a whole series of learning tasks related to diagnosis, treatment, and maintenance of relationships with patients. Gaining competency in these underlying strategies is a prerequisite to effective application in problem-based learning and must be addressed as part of the formal medical school curriculum.

It is important to differentiate training in these strategies from simply offering students the opportunity to engage in problem solving. Neglecting to teach and learn these underlying strategies, and simply having students solve medical problems (which is the current status in most medical schools), is analogous to requiring that the cranial nerves be remembered without training in the skill of active memorization (which, unfortunately, is also the current status in most medical schools).

One cannot assume that students have mastered these learning strategies for problem solving in their long history of education, or that they will *pick them up* in the context of clinical problem solving. As Crutchfield (1969) states: "Productive thinking and problem solving are complex processes which require direct attention in and of themselves" (p. 54). The strategies of clinical problem solving initially must be introduced and practiced on their own. Only after the learner has mastered, and can differentiate among, these strategies should there be a gradual and purposeful integration of medical content which reinforces the application of specific strategies and fosters their generalization (transfer). The sequential *learning strategies* which must be internalized are: (1) recognizing a problem; (2) generating conditional hypotheses; (3) characterizing the problem; (4) formulating a solution; (5) deciding on a solution; and (5) assessment of results.

Characterizing a problem involves several discrete activities which must be understood and practiced. First, a problem must be *recognized.* This important and creative step is often neglected in traditional problem-based learning curricula which typically provide *ready-made* problems to be solved. In reference to this oversight, Crutchfield (1969) states:

> This crucial stage in the productive thinking process tends to be short-circuited or completely omitted in the typical problem solving. . . . The relevant terms and conditions of the problem are clearly and specifically stated, and the question to be answered is explicitly put. (p. 59)

In your future medical practices, you will not be given problems to solve by your patients but rather will be required to recognize vaguely implied or presented symptoms and signs which must be sorted out. The *chief complaint* written on the patient's chart typically is only part of the patient's *problem.* You must *learn* to actively search for the patient's problems with the help and cooperation of the patient him/herself. This search must focus on the whole patient. You are often only *taught* to define part of the problem, typically the organic aspect, and this can lead to failure to recognize its complexity (e.g., psychological and sociocultural aspects).

In a broad and very real sense, failing to learn how to uncover and recognize patients' problems not only will inhibit your abilities to help individual patients but also will inhibit your abilities to advance medicine beyond the status quo. Medicine requires great problem-solving skill in uncovering and recognizing new diseases as soon as they emerge. As demonstrated in the AIDS pandemic, expediency in the recognition and definition of new diseases is essential to an effective response.

Problem recognition involves both cognitive and affective elements. Cognitively, problem recognition is a result of perceived discordance or contradiction between two or more *pieces* of knowledge (e.g., the patient's description of chest pain is inconsistent with the presence of a healthy heart). In a physician-patient interaction this knowledge may include the physician's prior medical knowledge, information gained from the patient's chart, or the patient's physical condition/appearance, behavior, and history. From this analysis of problem recognition, we can see the importance of previously described learning skills related to gathering and encoding information (e.g., memorization, bodily-kinesthetic skills).

However, we can also see that the presence of these skills is *necessary but not sufficient* to implement problem recognition. It is the ability to identify contradiction or discordance which characterizes this strategy. Although a solid knowledge base (built through reading and remembering), good communication, physical exam and observational skills are prerequisites for problem recognition, specific learning and strategy development exercises for problem recognition should focus on the ability to recognize contradiction, dissonance and discrepancy.

The affective side of problem recognition is having both a *sensitivity to,* and the *excitement* that is derived from, the experience of contradiction or discordance. Problems are viewed as challenges rather than impediments or hurdles. A second important affective element of problem recognition involves a healthy *skepticism* or doubt related to the perceived world. This skepticism extends to *authority* and *expertise* in defining this world. Finally, these affective states must be combined with another, or a positive self-perception or *self-confidence.*

At one level, problem recognition may involve uncovering a contradiction in the data and daring to challenge *accepted views* where diagnoses and treatment options are considered. At another level this may include persistence in trying to uncover the patient's hidden agenda or, together with the patient, identifying the patient's *chief concern.* Students with a history of early educational experiences which promote the cognitive and affective elements of problem recognition will have an advantage. However, all of these important cognitive and affective components of this strategy can and should be developed and fostered in medical school by students, faculty and the administration.

Although problem recognition is the crucial first step, its cognitive and affective elements reappear continuously throughout the problem-solving process. After all, new information is constantly being gathered and encoded, some of which may contradict previous findings. This leaves the door open for new problems to be recognized.

To develop the cognitive and affective features of problem recognition, review case histories with an open mind and a discerning eye. Rather than waiting until the end to formulate a definition of the problem, continually check for contradictions and discrepancies throughout. Consider the following example. What is the patient's problem? Why is she in your office? What are your diagnostic impressions and the perceived contradictions between the information and your line of thinking after paragraph #1, #2, #3? What is the *relevant* information?

The patient is a 47-year-old woman, married, with two children ages 24 (married and away) and 16 (lives at home). She presents with headaches for the last three months. They seem to be bilateral and toward the back of the head. She describes them as a *knot* in her head. She has been under a lot of pressure at work and her 16-year-old has been difficult to manage at home. Her husband is not much help around the house.

She feels that the headaches have *zapped* her energy. She uses the following expressions: "I have no energy to do anything"; and "I can't even get out of bed in the morning." She does not maintain eye contact and sighs at points in the interview. She reports that she's feeling very moody and withdrawn. Her appetite is very poor.

She eats a little and very slowly. In spite of this she has gained some weight recently (125 to 128 lbs.). The following lab test results are available: CPK = 540; Triglycerides = 192; SGOT = 54.

This example illustrates the complexity and dynamic nature of problem recognition throughout the encounter and the subsequent reporting of lab results. As more information is gathered (emotional, physical, and biochemical) we view the presenting problem, first in light of emotional functioning, and then in light of physical functioning. Recognizing and sorting through these areas is the essential first step in problem solving. Generating tentative hypotheses is the next strategy in problem solving. In the previous example, we begin by generating hypotheses related to stress, then depression and finally thyroid function.

In research this step is referred to as generating conditional hypothesis. In attributional research, it is making causal inferences and sorting them out from conditional relationships (those events or behaviors which are not causally but rather associatively related). Elstein et al. (1972) state that this strategy often occurs in clinical problem solving after only a few cues have been provided and before clinical data has even been gathered. These cues could include information from patient charts, previous medical knowledge, appearance of the patient, previous knowledge of the patient, etc. The process of generating clinical hypotheses escalates with perception of the patient's chief complaint. Regarding the strategy of hypothesis generation, Elstein et al. (1972) state:

> The components are: attending to initially available cues; identifying problematic elements from among these cues; associating from problematic elements to long-term memory and back, generating hypotheses and suggestions for fur-

ther inquiry; and informally rank-ordering hypotheses according to the physician's subjective estimates. (p. 89)

At this point in the problem-solving process a condensed version of the more formal strategies used in the solution weighing and decision-making step described below are implemented to ensure that the potential solutions are at least *in the right ball park*. It is imperative that learners be given the freedom to explore, and the freedom to fail, during this step. It is this feeling of freedom which supports travel down creative paths. The following exercises can be employed to develop and refine your ability to generate tentative hypotheses based on the available cues. Use the exercise with each of the practice cases below:

Exercise

In each of the two vignettes below, identify the relevant cues and define your initial conditional hypotheses. Examine the facts of each case. For each *fact* considered *separately*, list 2 or 3 hypotheses. Afterward make a list of all hypotheses relevant to the facts considered *together*. Compare the lists. Look for omissions. Ask yourself if other potential (even *far-fetched*) solutions exist. Rate all hypotheses on the basis of plausibility, interest, and familiarity to you. Notice the similarities and differences in your ratings, and think of the implications for problem solving.

Case 1   The patient is a sixteen-year-old female who told the receptionist that her mother brought her in for a routine physical exam. Vital signs are normal. Mother stated that she has been *tired* and missed school. She reported to the nurse that she has gained four pounds in the last two months.

Case 2   The patient is a forty-two-year-old male whose complaint is chest pain. He stated on the questionnaire that his occupation is an air traffic controller and that he has a family history of heart disease. You meet him going into the exam room, he left "to go outside for a smoke."

The next step is to characterize the problem or to gather new information and use knowledge (information which has been gathered using reading, note-taking, and communication skills, and stored in memory) to address the potential or conditional hypotheses defined. New information is generated from observation (e.g., perception) and manipulation (e.g., communication) of the problem field. Using knowledge implies searching for similarities and differences between new information about the problem and previous knowledge. This strategy highlights the importance of gathering (e.g., spatial perception) and storing (memorizing) information in accessible *compartments*. Accessible means generalizable to many problems based upon their underlying characteristics.

During this step, you are differentiating and integrating characteristics of the new problem situation with characteristics of previously encountered problems or with general principles and categories of knowledge. An important aspect of this process is discriminating between what is, and what is not, relevant to the present problem from the information gathered. This would include identifying inferences and assumptions and removing possible sources of bias. In the example above, we may think we know how and why hypothyroidism presents, but we must question these assumptions and be ready to see this as a unique patient with different characteristics. In this regard, Crutchfield (1969) warns us about another potential problem with structuring problem-based learning exercises:

> In the highly structured problem exercises . . . the problem information is substantially "predigested" for the student; the problem conditions are rigorously specified, the relevant facts are clearly stated, and all irrelevant facts are omitted. (p. 61)

In cases where problems are presented, care should be taken to ensure that the student will learn to observe, retrieve, differentiate, and integrate relevant from irrelevant information and cues. These are learning strategies integral to clinical problem solving which need to be practiced in relation to this skill.

Controlling inferences is an important strategy during the process of gathering information. This involves learning how to make *accurate* inferences and to recognize those not-so-accurate inferences that we automatically make. Information gathered from history (symptoms), and exam (signs), is always complemented by *implicit* information or data which we generate or create ourselves in response to this input. This *implicit information* is the product of inference. An example of an inference would be:

> You ask your new patient how things are going at home; she responds that Johnny has been sick and that has meant a loss of income for the family and his grades are declining. If you don't already know, you might infer that Johnny is her son; that he has been missing school; that she (or her husband) had to stay

home from work; that because he has been out of school, he has missed important learning, and/or failed to make up assignments; etc.

Often we do not even distinguish between information actually gained through gathering and encoding, and the inferences we make to fill in the gaps. Johnson-Laird and Wason (1980) cite research which suggests that the ability to make inferences is a strategy which can be learned and which is important for not only problem solving but for effective reading and memorizing as well. In this regard, Nickerson (1986) states:

> . . . good readers are more likely than poor readers to build a representation of the events in a story from which inferences can be made. Moreover, the building of such a representation itself requires the making of implicit inferences from the information that is explicitly contained in the story. Having such a representation, one is in a better position to interpret further information in the story and to integrate it with what one already knows. (p. 347)

Inferences are often unconsciously made in the direction of a favored line of thinking or hypothesis. This *inference bias* is extremely important to recognize in the clinical problem-solving process. Nickerson (1986) refers to it as confirmation bias which "is a bias toward interpreting data as being more supportive of a favored hypothesis than they actually are" (p. 356). You must learn to recognize and reduce this bias by making accurate and objective inferences from the data at hand.

Nickerson (1986) distinguishes between two types of problems: closed and open-ended. Closed problems have a prescribed set of inferences which lead to one correct solution. Open-ended problems, on the other hand, may have many sets of inferences (or paths) and more than one appropriate solution.

In medicine, one will be confronted with both closed and open-ended problems to solve. First it is important to learn to differentiate between the two types of problems. It is also important to become proficient in controlling and generating inferences for both types of problems. Consider the following examples:

> *Case 1*   A ten-year-old girl, with whom you are familiar, presents with a fever (temp 101°), diarrhea, and a non-productive cough of 2 days duration. From your knowledge of the family, you infer that she has not travelled abroad recently nor contracted a parasitic condition at home. Upon a brief physical you conclude that she has the flu and that plenty of liquids, rest and a cough suppressant would be in order. You infer that the patient contracted the virus from a family member or classmate, and

that it will run its course if the patient can stay comfortable, hydrated and maintain a strong immune response.

Case 2 A forty-two-year-old salesman presents with stomach pains for the last month. He describes it as a dull pain which is aggravated by spicy food, and alleviated by antacids. He has not noticed changes in his stool. He reports that he is under extreme pressure to sell. He drinks up to 10 cups of coffee in the morning, and often drinks alcohol during lunch with clients and reluctantly reports having 'Maalox cocktails' (Maalox and scotch whiskey mix) to alleviate the pain and sleep. You infer that the patient is having gastric pain which is aggravated by alcohol and caffeine. You infer that it might be difficult for him to make all of these life-style changes at once and that it might be best to begin with one change and to establish a plan with the various strategies and timetables for each other necessary change.

It is important to recognize which type of problem you are dealing with and to modify your approach accordingly. Often medical students and practicing physicians approach open-ended problems as closed problems. In Case 2, for example, the focus could have been on relieving stomach pain through medication and not dealing with life-style factors.

Making inferences is a necessity. Physicians do not have the time to ask about *everything* and patients do not have the time or patience to answer *all* questions. However, it is important to remember that making too many inferences when collecting important information diminishes accuracy in problem solving. Checking the number, appropriateness and accuracy of inferences is an extremely important strategy in learning how to problem solve. Read the following verbal exchanges and identify and consider the accuracy of the inferences.

Physician: So what have you been taking for the headaches?
Patient: Aspirin.
Inference: Regular strength; two every four hours.

Physician: How long have you been taking the aspirin?
Patient: About a week, I guess.
Inference: 7 days; every day.

Physician: How has that worked?
Patient: Okay for a little while.

Inference: **The pain goes away right after aspirin but comes back within an hour.**

As the example illustrates, making inferences has a lot to do with what one learns in a problem-solving encounter. It is important to recognize and check one's inferences for accurate clinical problem solving. To become an effective problem solver, you must learn to *effectively* make inferences. A curriculum which is designed to teach medical students how to gather information to problem solve must teach this basic learning strategy.

Another important strategy for characterizing a problem is defining implications. If previous knowledge has been learned with meaning, then the development of these implications will be enhanced. Defining implications means characterizing the complaint or problem in more than a simplistic, objective fashion. It means *assessing the value* of the information obtained. For example, it means more than simply *the patient is homeless*. It means that *the patient is homeless and most likely unable to pay for expensive medication and also will have difficulty complying with a regular regimen; therefore, I will attempt to manage the problem accordingly.* Forcing yourself to define the *implications* of characteristics of the problem will enhance your ability to develop appropriate cues.

Another strategy for characterizing a problem appropriately is to monitor *interference* which may be created by previous problem-solving activities. Barrows (1985) alludes to the positive influence of previous problem-solving activity. He states:

> Retrieval and use of information in the task context, in medicine the clinical context, requires that the information is learned in work with patients and their problems, so that the cues that appear while working in the task situation will stimulate retrieval of the appropriate information through memory associations. Learning in a clinical context causes the information that is being acquired to be organized or structured in the mind in ways that are useful to clinical tasks. (p. 4)

One's perception and analysis of the current problem, however, can also be skewed or biased by previous problem-solving activities. According to Vinacke (1952), this is due to "resonance" in which solutions to current problems are sought by looking for specific cues in memory of previous problems (p. 174).

This bias may influence the recognition and characterization of the problem, as well as subsequent strategies (selection of analytic methods, range of possible solutions, etc.). Thus, learning problem solving only within the context of specific problems may create a situation in which *resonance* continually interferes with the problem-solving process. It is especially important in medicine that you learn the importance of the unique perspective of each patient, and that this perspective be analyzed and considered in the generation of solutions tailored to that patient's problem. The strategy of monitoring interference includes continually asking yourself how the current problem might *differ* from problems to which you find yourself comparing it. This includes viewing the patient and environment in a different light and observing the unique manifestations (viz., signs, symptoms) of the disease and illness. Remember that clinical problem solving involves recognizing and characterizing a problem from a very complex set of circumstances. The solution always requires that one be able to sort through complex and important relationships among variables.

Some problem-based learning curricula, contrary to intent, may be perpetuating *rote* learning of problems and solutions thereby generating disruptive resonance by prematurely tying general principles to specific contextual elements of a problem. At the same time they are at fault for and not equipping students with learning strategies to investigate every problem as a unique set of circumstances. As Vinacke (1952) states: "In order to solve a problem, it is necessary to utilize objects in new ways or to reorganize the elements of a situation" (p. 175). It is important for the learner to develop both a knowledge base with particular emphasis on *generalizability of underlying principles* and the analytic skills necessary to solve problems. These two components must initially be differentiated in teaching and learning to minimize the intrusive efforts of *signals* linked to solving previous problems. Because resonance ultimately will play a role once the learner begins to solve problems and will continue throughout his/her career, he/she must learn to recognize its presence and remain unbiased in analysis of the current problem situation.

Once the problem has been fully characterized, the next step is to narrow your working hypotheses (viz., differential diagnoses) to a minimum by turning to other sources of information to help in the decision-making process. This might include questioning the patient about related issues such as family, past health, etc. (communication skills), and gathering data from physical examination and/or laboratory tests (observation skills).

During this step of ruling out hypotheses, one is constantly using another important strategy in problem solving: the strategy of *decision making.* This involves: (1) assigning value to potential outcomes (evaluating); (2) assessing the likelihood of outcomes (determining probabilities); (3) estimating the reliability and validity of information (both currently gathered and present in previous knowledge); and (4) eliminating or confirming hypotheses. The first three steps in decision making often occur intuitively and without formal consideration. However, it is important when learning problem solving to systematically consider each step.

In clinical problem solving, assigning value to outcomes involves prioritizing potential diagnoses in terms of their potential impact on the patient. In this regard, it is common practice to *rule out* life-threatening problems immediately. It is then important to consider the potential *value* of diagnosing other conditions in the problem list or differential.

As you consider the value of specific diagnoses it is important to consider, at the same time, the probability of their occurrences. In this regard it is clear how problem solving should proceed when value and probability are both high, but what if value is high and probability is medium or low? Resolution would depend on the value and probability of other potential diagnoses and contingency factors such as time, cost and outcome of the third step in decision making: estimating reliability and validity of information.

Often during learning it is important to exaggerate the uniqueness of each of these steps to ensure that they are used during decision making. A helpful exercise is to assign a rating (one to ten) for value and probability and for the reliability/validity of supporting information (Kassirer & Gorry, 1978). You can keep a record of your ratings for each patient that you see. Compare your scores with the final outcomes of diagnosis and treatment. Modify your ratings as necessary.

The final step involves eliminating or confirming diagnoses in the differential. Kassirer and Gorry (1978) define a confirmation strategy as "that with which the clinician tried to prove a hypothesis by matching characteristics of the disease or clinical state under consideration" (p. 249). They defined an elimination strategy as the use of "questions about findings that are so often found with a given disease that their absence weighs heavily against the hypothesized disease" (p. 249). These two strategies are continually used from the time the first hypothesis is generated and are not always implemented sequentially. It is important to *elicit* information which will confirm or eliminate hypotheses and also to *review* the findings in light of their potential confirming and eliminating power. Use the following exercise to apply the steps of decision making in considering your hypotheses or differential diagnoses.

Exercise

Consider Case 1 (ten-year-old girl with fever, diarrhea and cough) and Case 2 (forty-two-year-old salesman with stomach pain) which were used to practice controlling and generating inferences. With the limited amount of information that you have, how would you answer the following questions?

- In each case, what diagnoses do you want to rule out immediately?
- What are the *values* of potential outcomes or diagnoses in each case?
- What is the likelihood of each?
- How reliable (*trustworthy*) and valid (*truth-telling*) is your data?
- What additional information would you need to *eliminate* or *confirm* important diagnoses being considered?

The final step in problem solving is systematically analyzing and assessing the adequacy of the chosen solution to your problem. This step does not include new learning strategies but rather the same strategies used in the first steps: recognizing discordance, skepticism and doubt, identifying assumptions and bias, checking inferences, formulating and testing hypotheses, confirming and eliminating hypotheses, etc. During this step, however, the entire process is performed deductively rather than inductively. You begin with the solution and work backward through the steps to the original problem-recognition strategy. Along the way, implementation of specific strategies is checked for clear thinking and thoroughness.

It is important to note that this problem-solving process, which has been described in a systematic and sequential manner, does not often occur so precisely in real life. In fact, problem solving most often begins in the middle and its end is not clearly demarcated. As Crutchfield (1969) states:

> Typically, the stages [of problem solving] are overlapping and intertwined. The process does not necessarily begin at the beginning and end at the end. Often an idea occurs to the person before he has adequately stated the problem; a period of information processing may precede rather than follow the emergence and formulation of a problem; an answer may wander in search of an appropriate question. There may be direct insightful leaps from problem to solution with the intervening steps of logical thought not filled until after the fact. (p. 64)

It is, however, important to learn and follow the steps and apply the strategies in the logical sequence described. It is also important for the experienced clinical problem solver to *check* the problem-solving process for missing steps and strategies which may result from habit and inattention. Remember that these steps and learning strategies underlie all problem-solving situations. In addition to formulating a clinical diagnosis, the process can be applied to defining a treatment and management plan, adopting life-style change to prevent disease, etc.

COMMUNICATION SKILLS

Interpersonal Perception

Observational skills apply to interpersonal as well as spatial relations. As medical students you must develop skills which enable you to learn from observing interactions between care seekers and significant others (e.g., mother and child, husband and wife). In addition, you will learn a great deal about a patient and his/her problem by observing the patient's behavior with you.

Like spatial perception, interpersonal perceptual skills include establishing meaning and using description. There is, however, one marked difference in the character of these skills. Interpersonal perception relies more on your personal expectations. Recognizing and modifying (if necessary) expectations are important strategies for improving interpersonal perception.

Three types of interpersonal expectations have particular relevance to clinical problem solving: category-based, target-based and normative. The first, *category-based expectancies*, "reflect certain presumptions about groupings in our society and are not richly informed by individuating facts" (Jones, 1990, p. 5). You begin to form *category-based expectancies* when you preview the patient's chart *before* the actual interaction. The patient's age, gender, ethnicity (as reflected in the last name), designation as a first-time patient, and complaint all represent the *raw material* for the formation of this type of expectation. Much like the strategies identified for improving reading, memory, and spatial perception, expectancies represent our need as human beings to organize and group input stimuli. As we have seen in the discussion of problem solving above, these categorical expectancies generally interact with knowledge about the presenting complaint to serve as the basis for early hypotheses formation.

The most extreme form of category-based expectancies, negative stereotype, is extremely important to recognize and modify. These stereotypes generally "involve distortion and oversimplification" and are "tenaciously held and quite resistant to the implications for change of any new information" (Jones, 1990, p. 89). Not all stereotypes are *extreme*, but they often inhibit clinical problem solving (e.g., a female patient in her forties complaining of mood swings is experiencing menopause).

In most instances category-based expectancies are combined with, and supplanted by, *target-based* expectancies (Jones, 1990). The latter are tied directly to your experience with the patient, begin formation during the first interaction, and will continue to be refined throughout your relationship with the patient. These are the expectancies that are based upon our previous encounters with and knowledge about the patient (Jones, 1990).

The strategies of recognizing and refining target-based expectancies are guided by certain assumptions. First, as you might expect, it is more difficult to *accept* disconfirming information about target-based expectancies than about category-based expectancies. In addition it is important to recognize that there is a tendency to give more validity to *first impressions* over recent experience if the two conflict in the formation of target-based expectancies. The old saying that first impressions are everything is not far from the truth and should be considered carefully in relation to the development of interpersonal perception learning skills related to interpersonal perception.

A helpful exercise is to identify and list the category and target-based expectancies you have for the next person (or patient) you meet. Assess the validity of these expectancies as well as their strength in forming your perception of the individual. How would they influence your clinical problem-solving and patient education behaviors? How would they influence your relationship with this patient? Return to the list of expectancies the next time you interact with this individual. Reassess your perception and modify it if necessary. Become aware that this process always takes place, most often at a subconscious level.

The third type of expectancy relates to your, and the patient's, role and behaviors in the context of the doctor-patient interaction. These are called *normative expectancies* (Jones, 1990). In a problem-oriented interview, a patient is *expected* to provide a chief complaint, answer questions which characterize the complaint and agree to be examined physically. A patient who refuses to answer questions or one who expresses seductive behavior violates normative expectancies. A strategy in developing interpersonal perceptual skills is to learn to recognize normative expectancies and their antitheses, check their validity, and assess their impact on communication and problem solving in the interaction.

To practice this strategy, make a list of the behaviors you expect to observe in the next person (or patient) you will encounter. Check this list against the actual behaviors observed. How did these behaviors, or lack thereof, influence the interaction?

Appearance cues are another important source of interpersonal observational data which you gather in order to learn from the patient (Jones, 1990). Attending to these cues is much the same as attending to structural aspects of spatial relations. Categories of size, shape, and relationship to the environment are all important appearance cues in interpersonal perception. Consider your personal (valuative and emotional) responses to the following appearance cues in people (or patients) you meet for the first time:

Size	*Shape*	*Relationship*
Tall	Neat	Young
Short	Disheveled	Old
Thin	Clean	Aloof
Fat	Untidy	Attentive

How could your valuative and emotional responses influence your interaction with a patient?

Appearance cues are often a source of bias and stereotype. They are powerful elements of interpersonal perception, and recognition of their presence and impact is an important aspect of the observational skill of interpersonal perception.

Beyond initial expectancies and cues, interpersonal perception becomes directed toward perception of the other's verbal and nonverbal behavior within the interaction. Effective observation of nonverbal behavior includes attention to *changes* in appearance, such as *becoming more fidgety* or *maintaining less eye contact.* Attending to these changes in appearance as they relate to what you and the patient are saying is an extremely important aspect of learning about the patient's problem.

Interpreting emotions is an important strategy of interpersonal observation (Jones, 1990). Observation can tell us much about a person's emotional status. If the patient is smiling, she could be happy. If she fails to make eye contact and sighs often, she may be sad or depressed.

Physical behavior, however, can be misleading. A patient who is smiling and apparently happy may be in denial, an early stage of grief. Medical students, who are expected to become expert diagnosticians with patients whose problems almost always involve emotions, should develop skills in learning how to interpret emotion from physical behavior and to check those interpretations using communication skills when necessary. Jones (1990) states:

> Students of person perception **should** be able to say something about how emotions are revealed even when the person experiencing the emotion is attempting to conceal it. This is, after all, one of the skills that we normally associate with the gifted therapist, the shrewd diagnostician, and those "untrained" people around us who seem especially deft at penetrating the disguises and masks of others. (p. 20)

Observation of verbal behavior involves listening. Although similar in some respects to the strategy of listening during note-taking, the difference lies in its interactive nature. In both contexts, listening is attending to the verbal behaviors of the other. In the clinical interaction, behaviors which you can use both to improve the strategy of listening and to convey to the patient that you are listening include verbal following, summarizing and paraphrasing.

Verbal following means connecting to the other's last statement. For example, when the patient says, "The pain has been getting worse and I'm really scared," a statement like, "It sounds like it's been a difficult time for you; could you tell me what scares you?" is a good example of verbal following.

Summarizing is the essence of describing what the other says in a capsulated form. Summarizing has many benefits for the interviewer. First, it helps sharpen listening by forcing one to attend to details. This can improve the problem-solving process and facilitate the immediate memory of both you and the patient. For example, by listening to yourself summarize the information you obtained about the history of the present illness, you may realize you omitted a question about location of the pain. Also, as he listens, the patient may realize what *he really meant* was the pain was dull, *not* sharp. In addition, summarizing conveys to the other that you are listening. In this connection, it is important to always use as many of the patient's *own words* as possible. An additional advantage of using summary to learn about the patient's problem is that it facilitates subsequent memory of the interaction (viz., the strategy of rehearsal discussed under memorization above). In this regard, the use of summary can serve as an alternative to taking written notes during parts of the medical interview.

Paraphrasing is an abbreviated form of summary. It is essentially *restating* what the other says in a different way. Like summary, it is a verbal indicator to the patient that you are listening. Paraphrasing is an effective strategy for prompting the patient to continue talking on a topic.

Eliciting Information

Effective elicitation skills in the one-to-one doctor-patient encounter involve using information previously gathered to gain new information. From this perspective, the skill of eliciting information in a clinical interaction begins with questioning but then involves the use of skills previously mentioned, such as *listening* and *memorizing*, to then provide feedback to the patient in order to elicit more information. This *cyclical nature* of eliciting information is repeated often throughout the clinical interview as a means for learning about the patient and his/her problem.

The primary strategy for eliciting information is *questioning*. Questions can be more or less open or closed. Open questions give patients freedom in their responses. They also encourage the patient to be actively involved in the interview process and to maintain a great deal of responsibility for the content and direction of the interview. Open questions invite the patient to explore further; to expand and to elaborate upon a thought or feeling. They typically begin with *what, how,* and *could.*

Closed questions are appropriate in instances where you know more about the information that is needed. As such, they restrict the patient's responses and provide less opportunity for self-expression. They tend to encourage the patient to be passive, both in terms of the interview, and with respect to personal concerns about the illness. Closed questions help the patient focus when specific information is needed and typically begin with *is, are, do,* and *did.*

The sequence in which one asks questions is important. Generally this sequence *should proceed from open to closed* in relation to each content area (e.g., history of present illness):

Example:

> Open: "How would you describe the pain?"
>
> Closed: "Is it a sharp pain?"
>   "Where is it located?"
>   "How long have you had it?"

If you follow this sequence you can actually *save time* in your interview. In the above example, you may receive information from the patient about quality, location and chronology of the pain in response to your initial open-ended question. You thus have to ask fewer closed questions to receive information about the remaining characteristics of the chief complaint.

Another strategy for providing feedback for purposes of eliciting more information which relies most on your perspective is *interpretation.* An interpretation is one's verbally acknowledged *inference* of the feelings or thoughts underlying another's verbalization or action and is not to be confused with a diagnostic or etiological interpretation of physical symptoms. This strategy allows you to identify and label what you think the patient feels or thinks in order to clarify your perception with the patient. That is, the patient is provided with the opportunity to affirm, deny, or expand upon the interpretation as she/he sees fit.

Example:

> Doctor: "From what you've said about your pains, from the way your voice quivered as you spoke, it seems to me that you are very frightened by them."

Eliciting information also includes the strategy of *maintaining direction.* This involves managing the content and how it is presented in the interview. In a patient-centered interview, it is generally recommended that direction of the interview be *mutually maintained* by the patient and the physician. Frequent topic changes, non-contributory statements or questions, and *sidetracking* adversely affect the direction of the interview. Responding to the patient's preceding statements (e.g., "I understand, that must be difficult . . . ") and providing transitional statements (e.g., "Now I'd like to . . . ") can facilitate the direction in the interview. The ultimate goal of the interview is to gather the information in a logical, consistent and efficient manner necessary to help the patient. To effectively elicit information, each of these strategies plus selected strategies described above under listening and memorizing must be used.

Chapter 3

PLANNING SELF-DEVELOPMENT

The only man who is educated is the man who has learned how to learn; the man who has learned how to adapt and change; the man who has realized that no knowledge is secure, that only the process of *seeking* knowledge gives a basis for security. (Rogers, 1969, p. 104)

It is clear that we are living in a time when the validity of most knowledge, especially medical knowledge, is short-lived. Now, more than ever before, medical students must learn how to direct their own learning in the future. Learning how to learn independently not only leads to more effective learning after medical school, it can also result in more immediate learning successes during medical school. For example, research has demonstrated that medical students who take their basic science courses through independent study perform as well or better than those who take them through the traditional lecture-oriented curriculum (Stone, Meyer, & Shilling, 1991). Learning how to learn independently should complement classroom learning, thereby increasing students' academic performance during medical school and beyond.

Learning how to learn independently involves mastering all of the learning skills described thus far *plus* being able to *assess one's needs, define appropriate goals, objectives, and strategies to meet these goals and objectives, and to evaluate the successes and failures* which result from self-instruction. In this sense the learning skill of self-directed learning entails establishment of a structure or plan in which all of the learning skills previously discussed are *put into action.* Thus, self-directed learning *requires* the effective use of reading, memorizing, communication, etc., however, mastery of these skills alone is not *sufficient.* There is an additional requirement of developing and implementing an appropriate *plan* or structure for learning.

The structure of self-directed learning, like all of educational planning and implementation, mirrors that of clinical problem solving. Figure 17 outlines and compares these processes.

The first task to be accomplished is needs assessment. A major assump-

	Step 1	Step 2	Step 3
Self-directed learning	needs assessment	objectives/ methods	self-evaluation
Clinical problem-solving	diagnosis	treatment	follow-up

Figure 17. Comparison of self-directed learning and clinical problem solving.

tion of self-directed learning is that the adult learner can participate fully (not necessarily solely) in the assessment of his/her own needs. Often this can be accomplished subjectively by considering your own knowledge, skills or attitudes in relation to self-defined requirements. Other times, however, assessing your needs may require knowing how to *use outside resources* to help identify self-deficiency and/or the criteria for judging these needs. In both instances you must develop strategies which will enable you to perceive and define your strengths and weaknesses in knowledge, skills and attitudes.

Knowles (1980) states:

> The diagnostic process involves three steps: (1) the development of a model of desired behaviors or required competencies; (2) the assessment of the present level of performance by the individual in each of these behaviors or competencies; and (3) the assessment of the gaps between the model and the present performance. (p. 227)

The first step, defining the desired behaviors, can be accomplished by yourself or with the help of your peers or experts from research and teaching. Often students *skip* this important step and dive right into assessing current level of performance. Remember to take the time to define and *prioritize* the required competencies in any self-directed learning activity.

The second step requires that performance be assessed in relation to the specific level of concern (e.g., recall knowledge or demonstrate a skill). Often this can be accomplished with the aid of *old exams* or practice tests. It is important to remember to focus only on those questions, or sets of questions, which represent the prioritized areas. Sometimes oral quizzes by a study partner are effective in defining current performance levels.

The third step is to accurately define the differences between the first and second steps. It is answering the question: How much *more* do I have to know or be able to do?

The first strategy for learning how to routinely assess one's own learning needs is to *systematically approach* all experiences as potential learning experiences. Knowles (1975) states: "We must come to think of learning as being the same as living. We must learn from everything we do; we must exploit every experience as a learning experience" (p. 16). We must continually ask ourselves what knowledge, attitudes and skills *can I gain* from this experience and how can I use my learning skills for this purpose.

The second strategy is to approach each learning experience with the question: "What do I *really need* to know, be able to do, or appreciate?" As medical students you may expect that you need to learn more than you actually do. This expectation is often precipitated by unrealistic requirements defined by teachers and course coordinators. It is reinforced by a prevalent misconception of the unitary purpose of learning (i.e., to pass the next exam) combined with little time and training to *think* of personal needs. This strategy of prioritizing, then, is particularly difficult for many medical students. Without the experience of assessing and specifically defining one's needs, medical students often pass through training and are suddenly in their own *universities without walls* where they are expected to continue learning but cannot even begin because they cannot take this first step.

The second task in the process of self-directed learning is to develop clear learning objectives related to your needs and to identify methods of accomplishing them. This requires an understanding of the behavioral characteristics and levels of objectives, and the compatibility of learning methods. Part of choosing the appropriate learning methods is deciding which learning skill(s) to employ. Deciding to read will be an effective method of gaining knowledge, whereas it will be less effective in learning to communicate with patients (for a complete discussion of objectives and methods, see Chapter 7).

The next task in your self-directed learning experience is to evaluate your own performance. This involves the development of a plan for gathering usable, reliable and valid data on how well you have achieved previously defined criteria (see Chapter 7 for a complete discussion of evaluation of learning). This is basically the same as assessing your needs and completes the cycle of learning by bringing it back to the beginning.

Knowles (1975) elaborates on a specific strategy for practicing and accomplishing the skill of self-directed learning: the learning contract. It is a formal structure for planning and implementing the self-directed learning experience. Figure 18 presents an adaptation of Knowles' version of the learning contract with the addition of the critical feature of identifying and using appropriate learning skills for each learning objective.

LEARNING OBJECTIVES	LEARNING RESOURCES AND STRATEGIES	REQUIRED LEARNING SKILL(S)	EVIDENCE OF ACCOMPLISHMENT	CRITERIA AND MEANS OF VALIDATING EVIDENCE
STRUCTURE				
1. Define the molecular composition and consequences of complementary base pairing				
2. Identify characteristics of the double helix				
3. Recite experimental evidence supporting the role of DNA				
REPLICATION				
4. Explain the concept of semi-conservative replication				
5. Graphically define the mechanism of replication				
6. Identify replication enzymes				

Figure 18. Format of a learning contract.

To practice self-directed learning, complete the learning contract in Figure 18. Be as specific as possible. Next, develop a similar learning contract for taking a sexual history with a teenager of the opposite sex. Pay attention to the levels of objectives (i.e., knowledge, use of knowledge, attitudes, skills) and methods of learning that you define. How are your contracts similar? How are they different? Try developing and implementing a contract for something *you* are interested in learning.

Part II

THE TEACHER

INTRODUCTION

Medical education in the United States is undergoing the most profound reform since the introduction of the standardized four-year, two-step curriculum (two years in the basic sciences, two years in clinical rotations). Until recently, the emphasis has been on *differentiation of the disciplines* which has led to a focus on the accumulation and transmission of facts. The guiding principle of teaching has been (and still is in some arenas) to focus on the content of learning and to transmit this content as knowledge, often reduced to its essential elements within a disciplinary framework.

Curricular reform is grounded in a paradigmatic shift from the view that medicine is experimental science with an emphasis on parts (e.g., subspecialties) to "a systematic, integrated view of whole structures" (Bloom, 1992, p. 18). As described in Part I of this book, there is also a shift in our understanding of the nature of knowledge: most is short-lived and physicians-in-training must not simply learn new knowledge but also learn *how to acquire* and *use* new knowledge and skills. In other words, it is a conceptual shift from medical content to the process of learning. An essential feature of the reform is a shift in the role of the teacher from *purveyor of knowledge* to *facilitator of learning*.

Teachers of medicine must prepare their students to learn most effectively from their current environment while both in medical school and beyond. They must be able to help their students develop learning skills and to implement what are called *mediated learning experiences* (Nickerson, Perkins & Smith, 1985).

Part II of this book will describe the teacher's role in learner-centered medical education. In these chapters, the skills and strategies for *learner-centered teaching* will be presented and discussed.

It is important to recognize that although this book is divided into three parts, the topic—learner-centered medical education—should be viewed as a whole. In this regard, each part of the book is interdependent. To a great extent there is also a hierarchical relationship among the parts. That is, to understand and practice learner-centered teaching, one must build upon an understanding of learner-centered learning. Similarly, to structure a learner-centered medical school environment, one must understand both the concepts of learning and of teaching.

The teacher interested in learner-centered teaching must be thoroughly familiar with the concepts and strategies of learning presented in Part I. Practically speaking, there are many stated and implicit assumptions in the previous chapters which are important for teaching and will not be reconsidered. For example, how to prepare handouts which are organized to enhance memory and what to focus on when teaching problem solving will not be discussed. Hopefully, the astute teacher will be able to adopt these and many other suggestions and recommendations for teaching from the previous discussions of learning in Part I.

The purpose of Part II of this book is to expand our framework for understanding learner-centered medical education by viewing it from the perspective of teaching. What characterizes learner-centered medical education is its focus on learning skills or the *process* of learning. Teaching in a context where learning skills and the learner are emphasized means:

1. students are provided with the opportunity to apply skills from *each* level of learning to a subject area;
2. a developmental sequence or progression in the use of skills are followed such that the learner begins by increasing knowledge, learns to apply that knowledge (i.e., problem solve) and finally is able to create and work independently in the subject area. The sequence is important in that later skills incorporate (or build upon) previous skills;
3. differences in learning skills among students are respected; learning weaknesses are identified, problems are remediated, and strengths are reinforced;
4. teaching behaviors appropriately relate to the level of expected learning (flexibility in teaching behaviors is a requirement);
5. evaluation must focus on process (feedback offered to improve learning behavior) as well as outcome (judging the student's competence); and

6. a learning context is established in which learners perceive the value of what they are learning and thus are motivated to engage in the process.

The following chapters focus on each of these aspects of a learner-centered model of medical education. First, a teacher must recognize and appreciate differences in learning among students. Sometimes it involves identifying and remediating learning problems. With all students, teachers must be able to foster motivation and enthusiasm to learn. This is a prerequisite to planning and organizing an educational experience from a learner-centered perspective. Finally, and not least importantly, we will consider the teacher's interaction with the learner in the lecture, small group and individual tutorial contexts. Each of the chapters in this section will provide specific guidelines for teachers.

Chapter 4

RECOGNIZING AND REDUCING THE IMPACT OF INDIVIDUAL LEARNING DIFFERENCES

S ome learners will have an easier time than others mastering certain learning skills required in medical school. The reason, according to many educators, is variation in learning style. As we will see in this chapter, learning style represents a preferred way of learning, and the relationship between style and intelligence is a topic of great debate. The implications of the outcome of such a debate is reflected in, among other areas, concern about testing bias. In this regard, one learning style may be more conducive to learning and test-taking in the preclinical years and another in the clinical years of medical school.

Individual learning and testing differences could account for the low correlation between preclinical and clinical course grades, cited in the literature and the common, but largely intuitive, knowledge among faculty and administrators that certain students will excel in the preclinical years but not in the clinical years and vice versa.

There are many theoretical approaches to styles of thinking and learning described in the literature. All suggest that groups of people differ with respect to how they learn and their ability to master certain subject matter. The theorists would agree that it is important for learners to consider these differences when developing strategies for learning. They also would advocate attention to learning style in teaching and evaluation.

Two of the most respected and well-researched theories are Witkin's cognitive styles and Kolb's learning styles. They will be explored herein in terms of their implications for learning and teaching in medical school. In this chapter, you will learn to help students assess their style and to develop strategies for becoming *flexible* in the use of alternative styles. You will also learn to recognize and reduce the learning style bias inherent in your teaching methods, content and evaluation.

The concept of cognitive style was formalized by Witkin (cf., Witkin et al., 1977) who differentiated between learners who were more field-dependent and those who were more field-independent. Identification of cognitive style can be accomplished by testing for field dependence using the Group Embedded Figures Test (Witkin et al., 1971). Learners who are field independent will have a higher level of cognitive restructuring ability than their field dependent counterparts. As such, they will be better able to analyze, organize, and reorganize information and experience (Witkin & Goodenough, 1981; Davis, 1991). In contrast, the presence of strong field dependence indicates high interpersonal and communication skills.

It is evident that cognitive styles not only describe the student's approach to learning but also pervade other aspects of their psychological and social functioning such as personality and interpersonal skills. In this regard, field dependence is distinguished by greater reliance on, and attention to, other people in the environment. Research has demonstrated that:

> ... field-dependent people are more socially oriented, as shown, for example, by greater attentiveness to interpersonal cues, by a preference for being physically close to people and by a greater emotional openness in communication with others. In contrast, field-independent people have a more abstract, impersonal orientation. They are not usually very interested in others, and they show greater physical and emotional distancing. In sum, field-independent people seem to function with a greater degree of individual autonomy in their social-interpersonal behavior. (Goodenough, 1986, p. 7)

The implications of cognitive style for learning are dramatic. There is evidence to suggest that cognitive style may even play a role in determining your ability to develop learning skills. Many studies suggest that *field-dependent* as compared to *field-independent* learners are less efficient and less adept in many *traditional* academic learning tasks (Davis & Frank, 1979; Reardon et al., 1982; Cochran & Davis, 1987). These studies agree that when the volume of information to be processed is increased, field-independent learners have a distinct advantage. Davis (1991) summarizes these findings as follows: "The most consistent finding reflects that field-independent learners are more efficient than field-dependent learners, particularly in situations with higher information-processing demands" (p. 153). This would certainly imply an advantage for the field independent learner in much of the current preclinical curriculum.

Evidence is compelling that reading skills are related to cognitive style. Field-independent readers may be more proficient than field-dependent readers in reading comprehension and word recognition (Davis, 1991). This has been demonstrated with college populations as well as younger children. Because field-dependent readers may need more time to construct and process inferences, they also may have markedly lower reading speed rates (Cochran & Davis, 1987). This would suggest that cognitive style will also influence problem-solving abilities under *timed* situations. Greater proficiency in reading of field-independent learners may be related to increased attention spans among these learners (Berger & Goldberger, 1979).

There is also substantial evidence that the ability to memorize is influenced by cognitive style. Davis and Frank (1979) found that field-dependent learners had less efficient short-term memory processes. Other studies found that field-independent learners, relative to field-dependent learners, were significantly better at both short- and long-term memorizing (Davis, 1987; Davis & Cochran, 1987, 1989; Annis, 1979; Frank, 1983). Field-independent learners have demonstrated greater proficiency in recalling factual information from reading text (Spiro & Tirre, 1980) and listening to lectures (Frank, 1984). There is general agreement that field-independent learners' superior memorizing abilities derive from greater organizing and structuring abilities which are used to store and to retrieve information (Cochran & Davis, 1987; Davis, 1991).

According to Witkin et al. (1977), field-independent people are high in cognitive restructuring skills and low in social skills. Field-dependent people, on the other hand, are high in social skills and low in cognitive restructuring skills. Davis (1991) states: "Strengths of the field-independent learner were derived from their superior cognitive restructuring skills, whereas the strengths of the field-dependent learner were derived from their superior social skills" (p. 150).

Spatial perceptual ability also seems to be related to cognitive style. A variety of experiments have demonstrated that field-dependent people are much more dependent on the visual context or *field* in determining the nature of objects. They have greater difficulty interpreting and understanding objects that are detached from their natural and familiar surroundings. Of course, the implications of this for learning in medical school are far-reaching. One would immediately foresee difficulty in anatomy, histology, pathology, pathophysiology and other courses and clerkships which rely heavily upon visualizing body parts and structures outside of their natural contexts.

In keeping with these findings on spatial perceptual differences, Witkin et al. (1977) determined that medical students, as a group, have high spatial abilities. Another study found differences in spatial ability (as measured by cognitive style) among practicing physicians from different specialties (Goodenough et al., 1979). Radiologists and surgeons were significantly more *field independent* than were internists and psychiatrists.

Research has demonstrated that medical students, as a group, are more often field independent than field dependent. As a measure of self-selection, this finding is consistent with findings of other researchers that field-independent learners do better in science than field-dependent learners (Raskin, 1986). One study found that college senior pre-meds were more field independent than other seniors and that those who ultimately enrolled in medical school were more field independent than those applicants who did not (Goodenough et al., 1979). This same study found that of the 140 male pre-meds, only 3 percent of the most field-dependent group ever finally enrolled in medical school (Goodenough et al., 1979).

Recent evidence suggests that field-dependent and field-independent learners may not be using different cognitive processes but the same processes with differential effectiveness (Davis & Frank, 1979). This would also suggest that learning skills related to these cognitive processes can be strengthened (viz., that field-dependent learners, though initially disadvantaged, could develop their memorization, reading and spatial perceptual skills). In this connection, Witkin and Goodenough (1981) state that although many people are *fixed* in their cognitive style (either field-dependent or field-independent), others are *mobile* or have characteristics of both which can be called upon.

Faculty should help students recognize their cognitive styles and provide the necessary guidance in learning skills development as outlined in Part I of this book. Strengthening students' learning skills related to *both* styles must be complemented by adapting teaching methods as well. In this regard, cognitive style has implications for *how* one learns more than *what* one is learning. Field-dependent learners (and teachers) tend to prefer more discussion-oriented learning activities, while field-independent learners prefer more impersonal activities (e.g., reading, traditional lecture). It is important for teachers to help students assess their cognitive styles and to formally build into the curriculum opportunities for *selecting* educational methods where appropriate.[1]

In the clinical teaching experience, a critical issue is the match between preceptor and learner style. Research demonstrates that congruence between the teacher's and the learner's cognitive style leads to *greater mutual acceptance.* In this regard, one study found that a field-independent teacher gave all the field-independent students in the class higher grades than were given to the field-dependent students. In another class, the field-dependent teacher gave all the field-dependent students higher grades relative to the field-independent students (Bertini, 1986).

There is a danger, however, in assuming that match between teacher and learner styles will lead to *better learning.* In this connection, Witkin et al. (1977) caution that a contrast in styles between some learners in the class and the teacher may make the classroom more lively and perhaps growth enhancing because of the diversity of viewpoints.

It is clear that much more research must be done on match of teacher and learner cognitive style. Witkin et al. (1977) advise that teachers must be flexible, that is, willing and able to shift teaching strategies and methods so that both learning styles are addressed. Similarly, one can assume that it is important for students also to expand their flexibility of cognitive style to enable them to learn the diversity of material in the preclinical and clinical years. As Witkin et al. (1977) state: "The development of greater diversity in behaviors within individuals seems as important an objective as the recognition of diversity among individuals" (p. 53).

There is a rising sentiment among researchers that flexibility and strengthening of style can be promoted and supported by adapting the curriculum. Ultimately, students will have strengths and weaknesses in certain areas related to style (e.g., field-independent learners will perform better at cognitive restructuring tasks in anatomy lab exercises, whereas field-dependent learners will do better at communicating and history-taking tasks). However, it is imperative that training (skills development focusing on weaker style) and educational support (varying teaching methods and teaching styles) be implemented to promote learner-centered medical education.

Kolb's (1981) experiential learning theory and schema for assessing and understanding learning styles is another profitable way of examining learning differences. He describes learning as a four-stage process. First, you have concrete experiences of the environment in which you exist. Second, you observe and reflect on these experiences. Out of this reflection comes the development of abstract interpretation and generalization. Finally, you test the *new* abstract conceptualizations and generalizations in *new* situations as they guide *new* concrete experiences. In this

connection, Kolb (1981) differentiates among four different abilities necessary for effective learning: (1) concrete experience abilities, (2) reflective observation abilities, (3) abstract conceptualization abilities, and (4)
active experimentation abilities. These four abilities closely parallel the
levels of learning skills presented in Part I of this book.[2]

Kolb's (1981) learning abilities can be viewed as polar endpoints of two
dimensions of learning. The first is the concrete-abstract dimension.
The second is the active-reflective dimension. According to Kolb (1981),
each of us develops a learning style with strength toward one pole on
each of these dimensions:

> Some people develop minds that excel at assimilating disparate facts into
> coherent theories, yet these same people may be incapable of or uninterested
> in, deducing hypotheses from those theories. Others are logical geniuses but
> find it impossible to involve themselves in active experience. (p. 237)

Using the Learning Style Inventory, which portrays the learning
dimensions on an *x and y axis,* Kolb (1976) has defined four different
styles. The *converger* has strengths in abstract conceptualization and
active experimentation. According to Kolb (1981), those who possess this
style are exceptional in the practical application of ideas. Research
demonstrates that convergers tend to be unemotional, would rather deal
with inanimate objects than other people, tend to have narrow rather
than global interests, and often specialize in physical sciences. As a
group, engineers tend to be convergers.

Divergers, on the other hand, are the learning opposites of convergers.
They are oriented toward concrete experience and observation. They
tend to be imaginative brainstormers who are emotional and interested
in people. This style is often found in students who major in the
humanities.

Assimilators are strong in abstract conceptualization and reflective
observation. They are interested in abstract thinking but not the practical implementation of theory. Instead, they value the precision and
soundness of theoretical propositions. This learning style is characteristic of basic scientists as opposed to applied scientists.

Finally, there is the *accommodator* who is the learning opposite of the
assimilator. Accommodators' strengths lie in concrete experience and
active experimentation. They tend to be very flexible in their orientation to problem solving and are risk-takers. In addition, research shows
that they tend to be trial-and-error problem solvers and to get their

information secondhand from others rather than rely on their own analytical abilities (Kolb, 1981).

Kolb (1981) differentiates types of knowledge structures and inquiry processes associated with the different disciplines and describes the importance of match between personal learning styles and the approach to learning inherent in that discipline. He noticed that as an advisor at the Massachusetts Institute for Technology (MIT), some students experienced "a distinct loss of energy and increase in confusion" when they realized they were not cut out to be engineers. He states:

> That disciplines incline to different styles of learning is evident from the variations among their primary tasks, technologies and products, criteria for academic excellence and productivity, teaching methods, research methods, and methods for recording and portraying knowledge. (1981, p. 233)

Kolb's findings would support the contention that medical students must be flexible in their learning styles and that teachers must foster the development of this flexibility. They are expected to learn material in many different disciplines which, as we have seen in our discussion of cognitive styles, demands strength in one or another *style*. If, in fact, Kolb (1981) is correct in stating that the majority of learners who ultimately choose medicine are very close to the center of the x and y axes, then one would expect that flexibility of learning styles is imperative to survive medical school.

While there isn't a precise one-to-one relationship between learning skills and styles, the following figure illustrates probable weaknesses in learning skills associated with Witkin's and Kolb's styles of cognition and learning. Teachers should help students identify their styles and provide opportunities within courses to strengthen their deficiencies in the associated learning skills.

Endnotes

1. In deciding the appropriateness of educational methods, one must also consider the types of objectives to be met. For example, it would be less effective and efficient to provide information (develop the learner's knowledge) in a small group discussion than a lecture, no matter what the cognitive styles of the learner. It may be an effective alternative to allow the field-dependent learner to read the information and have opportunities to *discuss* it in a group to enhance understanding.

2. Skills for gathering information and forming knowledge could be considered concrete experience abilities. Utilization of knowledge is similar to reflective observation and abstract conceptualization. Finally, discovery is much like active experimentation.

Witkin	Kolb	Learning Skills To Be Strengthened
	Diverger	• spatial perception
Field Dependent		• reading
	Accommodator	• memorizing
		• problem-solving
	Assimilator	• physical exam
Field Independent		• social perception
	Converger	• communicating with patients
		• history taking

Figure 19. Comparison of cognitive and learning styles with reference to learning skills to be strengthened.

Chapter 5

IDENTIFYING LEARNING PROBLEMS

A major premise of this book is that very little attention is paid to how students learn in medical school. If this is true, then one would expect that even less time is devoted to identifying, and accommodating to, medical students with special learning needs. Although students with special learning needs occasionally are identified by admissions committees prior to entering medical school, most are not. Generally, these students possess great intellectual strengths but also have a significant *learning weakness* which is exacerbated by the structure and/or content of medical school. This weakness impedes learning and decreases academic performance in related areas.

The intellectual strengths of these students with learning problems are evident in their academic achievements prior to entering medical school. Indeed, their medical school applications and academic records were of sufficient quality to merit acceptance. All of these students excelled academically in their college environments. In most cases only subtle evidence, if any, exists in records of previous academic performance of underlying potential impediments to learning in medical school. This evidence might include an unusually low reading score in comparison to the applicant's other scores on the MCATs. It might consist of an uncharacteristically poor grade in a geometry or geography course in comparison to other course grades in college. Perhaps it is the marked absence of English literature or other courses which demand proficiency in reading.

On the whole, however, these students with special learning problems had learned to cope, and to excel, in most academic areas. It is the rigor and extraordinary demand of the medical school curriculum with its *high volume, high density and high expectations* that provides the context for these learning problems to manifest and grow. As Taylor (1992) states:

> . . . the elemental curriculum combines the properties of both gases and of

crystals: like the former, it is intangible and difficult to contain, and it expands promptly to fill whatever space is available; like the latter, it grows by continuous accretion of substance from the surrounding medium. (p. 1436)

For a substantial number of medical students, learning problems are formed and shaped by the environment of the medical school.

Many of the once capable students who fall victim to the medical school environment because of its failure to accommodate individual learning differences and needs, surface as the focus of discussion at preclinical and clinical student promotion boards. They typically fail or receive marginal performance grades in those medical school courses which demand greatest use of the learning abilities in which they are deficient (e.g., anatomy course and spatial perceptual abilities). On the other hand, they may perform well in courses, or parts of courses, which demand greatest use of abilities in which they are proficient (e.g., biochemistry course and memorization abilities).

Not all students with these learning problems surface in this manner. There are those who *squeak by* academically and experience extreme anxiety or become depressed because they cannot meet their own and other's expectations for learning. Still others may be moderately affected by their learning problems, have to work harder to achieve less, and thus become disillusioned and lose their enthusiasm for learning, for medicine, or both. Some may ultimately withdraw from medical school. All of these individuals with impaired learning abilities never achieve full academic potential.

It is incumbent upon medical educators to help students recognize their learning problems and to modify the medical school environment by accommodating to their needs from both a teaching and an evaluation perspective. Students themselves, as well as faculty, can play a more active role in the identification and remediation of these problems if they are aware that they exist and are familiar with methods of screening and remediation.

There is historical evidence which suggests that medical students with learning problems who survived early academic training and medical education later achieved eminence in medicine. For example, Harvey Cushing, eminent brain surgeon and Pulitzer Prize winning biographer, and Paul Ehrlich, renowned German bacteriologist, both exhibited evidence of language disability (Accardo, Haake, & Whitman, 1989; Thompson, 1969). Arthur Conan Doyle and Carl Gustav Jung were dyscalculic (Accardo, Haake, & Whitman, 1989). These accomplished learning disabled individuals were able to overcome the obstacles to learning which their educational environments presented. It is likely, however, that other potential pioneers in medicine were unable to overcome these obstacles and thus never allowed to flourish.

The extent of learning disability among medical students and of services provided by medical schools to learning disabled students is not well documented in the literature (Faigel, 1992). In one of the few published studies, among medical students attending Marshall University, approximately five percent were found to be dyslexic (Guyer, 1987). None of these students had received a diagnosis of dyslexia prior to enrolling in medical school. In a study of more than one thousand first-year dental students, 5.3 percent were diagnosed as learning disabled (Garrard, Lorents, & Chilgren, 1972). This figure compares to a prevalence of up to ten percent in the general population (Accardo, Haake, & Whitman, 1989). These data are, by and large, based upon traditional definitions of learning disability.

In contrast to the traditional approach, I would argue that a learning problem should be defined *in relation to the expectations of the academic environment.* A learning problem is: *academic performance which is significantly below performance potential because of a specific affective, cognitive, or structural (experiential) difficulty which is exacerbated by the extraordinary demands of the environment.* Using this definition and based upon my experiences and research in this area, I would estimate that between fifteen and twenty percent of medical students have identifiable and often remediable learning problems at some point in their medical school experiences, which stem from affective, cognitive and/or structural sources.

The *affective source* of learning problems can be triggered by events which demand personal adjustment. Some students have difficulty handling these events, and this difficulty either directly or indirectly results in poor learning and/or poor performance during evaluation. Specific trigger events which are common to medical students include transition into medical school or clinical rotations (see Chapter 7), marital or relational difficulties, illness or death in the family, and grades on tests which are below expectations. Students can react to these events with anxiety, depression or stress which persists and is exacerbated by the demands of the curriculum and/or the personality of the student. These affective reactions often can result in learning problems related to motivation and memory.

The cognitive source underlies the more traditional types of learning problems. The most common is atypically low reading ability in relation to intellectual capacity. This is commonly referred to as developmental dyslexia (Aaron & Phillips, 1986). I would estimate that as many as half of students who fail or do very poorly in medical school do so because of inadequate reading ability in relation to reading expectations inherent in the medical school curriculum. As discussed previously, these expectations have been defined as unreasonable and without forethought (Taylor, 1992).

A problem rooted in cognition which underlies poor performance in courses such as anatomy, and rotations such as surgery, is impaired spatial perception. It is estimated that measurable spatial deficits are present in as many as one third of all medical students and that seven to ten percent have *severe* learning problems in this area (Rochford, 1985).

Another type of learning problem which often combines cognitive and affective elements is an inability to effectively communicate orally with others. Quite often cultural and language barriers are contributory factors. Learning problems in this area typically become evident during clinical clerkships or during preclinical courses in medical interviewing.

In addition to cognition and affect, a third source of learning problems which is most often neglected relates to an individual's inability to *structure* his/her experiences in the environment. This includes a student's inability to organize and control the learning process. Specific problems relate to managing time and maintaining effective study habits and study skills. A student's physical condition, including the presence of a physical disability or illness, can contribute to learning problems in this area. The physical demands of matriculation in medical school, including long hours to meet study requirements, and mobility required to and from learning settings (e.g., departments, wards, hospitals), often tax the physically disabled student and negatively impact upon the learning process.

In this chapter, learning problems associated with each of these three sources will be described and illustrated with real case examples. In addition, specific screening and remediation guidelines for students, faculty and advisors are presented.

AFFECTIVE SOURCE

Affective states which negatively impact upon learning vary according to prevalence and severity. Figure 20 presents a hierarchy of affective states with the accompanying learning problems most common to medical students. At the base of the hierarchy are those affective states which are most prevalent and generally have the least severe impact upon learning. At the top are those which are least prevalent but generally have the most severe impact upon learning and academic performance.

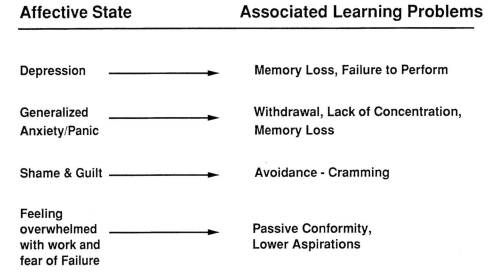

Affective State	Associated Learning Problems
Depression	Memory Loss, Failure to Perform
Generalized Anxiety/Panic	Withdrawal, Lack of Concentration, Memory Loss
Shame & Guilt	Avoidance - Cramming
Feeling overwhelmed with work and fear of Failure	Passive Conformity, Lower Aspirations

Figure 20. Hierarchy of affective states with commonly associated learning problems.

Feeling overwhelmed with schoolwork and fear of failure are the most common negative affective states experienced by medical students (Quirk et al., 1987). These feelings are evident in the following statements by students during structured interviews concerning their medical school experience:

> "I am seeing serious obstacles to overcome; that is coping with quantities of material in limited time purely to pass an exam."

> "The large amounts of facts that I did not retain [during preclinical courses] will hopefully not jeopardize my ability to perform [during clinical rotations]."

"I didn't think I learned enough in the first 2 years. . . . [There is] the anxiety of learning to make medical decisions. Always feeling you don't know enough and learning to live with that."

"I worry about harming or, God forbid, killing a patient."

"I expect it will be difficult—getting yelled at by superiors or being made to feel stupid."

In response to feeling overwhelmed and fearing failure, many students lower their academic aspirations to *simply passing tests*. This is reflected in the following representative quotes from students:

"I'm trying to lower expectations for myself so that I can try to be more content with my inadequacies."

"I just keep repeating *Pass = MD* . . . just as long as I pass."

"I'm used to being always fully prepared for whatever I have to do, and I'm starting to realize that I just can't do that if I want any enjoyment for myself at times."

Lowering aspirations potentially diminishes learning, stifles creativity and can result in a long-term negative attitude toward learning.

In addition to feeling overwhelmed and fearing failure, feeling shame and guilt are two affective states which are common among preclinical and clinical students. They are the antecedents of *fear of failure* when combined with lower than expected evaluations by self or other. Shame and guilt often represent emotional conflicts concerning academic performance and along with the preceding fear of failure manifest at the physical level in fatigue, headaches, eating disorders, etc. (Adsett, 1968; Thomas, 1976). At the psychological level, these emotions can diminish self-esteem and instill greater fear of failure (McMurray, Fitzgerald, & Bean, 1980; Quirk et al., 1987). During the preclinical years shame and guilt often result from the experience of not achieving one's expectations on course examinations. For some students this may involve failing an exam; for others with greater expectations, it may involve receiving an *average* grade. During the clinical years, these feelings often result from negative feedback from patients and attendings.

Shame and guilt often lead to avoidant learning behavior. Preclinical students who experience these emotions typically postpone (knowingly or unknowingly) studying subject matter in a course in which they are not achieving their expectations. Instead, they tend to focus on other courses, *extracurricular* activities, or interests unrelated to medical school. These students can develop associated problems with organizing their time and routinely end up *cramming* for exams. Clinical students who experience these feelings often will avoid being observed by preceptors and will not volunteer to act in emergency situations that involve patients and attendings. Some students who are seriously affected by these feelings may contemplate withdrawing from medical school and, in rare instances, take leaves of absence to engage in a medically related activity (e.g., medical research).

Consider the following student who developed avoidant learning behavior associated initially with fear of failure, and later with shame and guilt. As is often the case, this student had learning problems which may be considered secondary to those which are affective in nature. In most cases, a student who experiences these feelings and associated learning problems can be helped by faculty, advisors and administrators who identify the signs and symptoms and who work with the student to incorporate strategies which allow him/her to develop and maintain a feeling of control in the context of the learning environment. In addition, those administrators and faculty responsible for maintaining the academic environment should act to reduce the excessive volume of learning by *weeding out* less relevant material and fostering greater enthusiasm for learning (see Chapter 6).

Marie is a student from a top Ivy League college who entered medical school with superior qualifications. Her science G.P.A. was 3.3 and her MCATs were 12's and 13's in the sciences. In addition to these extraordinary academic achievements, Marie has many other talents. She is an accomplished musician and author.

During the first year of medical school she received satisfactory or near honors grades in all but one course.[1] During the summer after her first year, she was unsuccessful in her attempt to remediate her one marginal grade. Since students may carry one marginal grade and remain in good standing, Marie moved on to the second year of medical school. She began to fail or perform marginally in several courses. In the second semester of her second year, she decided to drop courses and extend her preclinical curriculum to three years. Also, at this time, she began to receive academic and psychological counseling.

Counseling revealed that during her first two years in medical school, Marie gradually became paralyzed by a fear of failure and ultimately internalized the negative evaluations. As the clinical years approached, she became even more concerned about her erratic preclinical performance. In an interview she stated: "Even worse, I'm afraid I'll hurt a patient because of [my] lack of knowledge." Her feelings of inadequacy and guilt were causing her to divert her attention from medical school to her other talents. This avoidant behavior contributed to further poor academic performance. A psychologist who evaluated Marie stated that she "seems frustrated with her studies . . . she is unsure where to begin and what information is most important."

Marie struggled with her problem and was eloquent in attempting to attribute cause and effect. In a letter she wrote:

> Although one could argue that I am incapable of earning higher marks in my medical courses, I believe that my stumbling block is an incurable ambivalence about being a medical student. One question this raises: is my ambivalence inherent to myself, or is my ambivalence due to medical school itself?
>
> . . . I must examine the extremes to which I have gone in order to avoid studying very carefully. Why have I been so consistently avoidant? I am not sure myself.

Finally, as a justification for taking a leave of absence she stated:

> My personal standards, while temporarily compromised, remain high enough to quit rather than settle for *good enough.*

As is typical of many students who experience this learning problem, she began her leave of absence by working in a medically related area of research.

Students with a history of low self-esteem and a high need for external reinforcement will experience more severe fear of failure or guilt due to poor performance. The commensurate learning problems of avoidance and withdrawal are likely to be exaggerated.

Anxiety is another affective state which potentially can lead to significant learning problems. It is a common reaction to test preparation (studying) and test-taking for a significant number of students. Many studies have shown that anxiety which is specific to the test-taking situation can negatively influence test performance (Alpert & Haber, 1960; Sarason, Mandler & Craighill, 1952; Mandler & Sarason, 1954; Howell & Swanson, 1989). Other studies suggest that some anxiety during test situations does not hinder test performance (Finger & Galassi, 1977; Spielberger, Anton & Bedell, 1976; Frierson & Hoban, 1987). All of these authors, however, would agree that excessive anxiety during testing is detrimental to both the student and to test performance. Few of these studies have examined the relationship between stress or anxiety and examination performance of medical students (Tooth, Tonge & McManus,

1989). One study assessed the relationship between test anxiety and performance of medical students on the NBME Part I Examination and found a significant relationship that students with low test anxiety performed better than those with moderate or high anxiety (Frierson & Hoban, 1987).

Test anxiety can occur in students in preparation for or during course exams, standardized tests (e.g., shelf exams, National Board exams) or other means of performance evaluation (e.g., performing a physical exam while being observed). In severe cases, the feelings of dread and anxiety are often accompanied by physical sensations such as excessive sweating, hot and cold flashes, dizziness, palpitations and choking. Test-taking anxiety may be associated with fear of failure or poor academic self-concept, but certainly not all students who experience these feelings react with anxiety (Howell & Swanson, 1989).

Learning difficulties associated with anxiety and panic include lack of concentration (in severe cases *blackouts*) and mental as well as physical withdrawal from the studying or test-taking situation (or from school). These difficulties are accompanied by a strong urge to flee the situation and feelings of dread. It is my experience that as many as 3 percent of medical students have intrusive test anxiety and are severely hampered in their learning and test-taking by this condition. Another 3 to 5 percent experience some test anxiety that negatively influences their well-being and academic performance.

Affected students as well as faculty and advisors can play important roles in identifying and defining the scope of the problem. In less severe cases, a faculty advisor can help the student by providing training in progressive relaxation techniques such as visual imagery, muscle tension relief and deep breathing. Often this limited training, combined with a commitment to change and independent practice of relaxation techniques, will help the student overcome his/her episodic anxiety. In the most severe cases the advisor or faculty member will most likely have to refer the student to the counseling center. Some of these students ultimately may require pharmacologic intervention combined with intensive behavioral training and psychotherapy.

Consider the case of William, who was referred to me for academic counseling by his faculty advisor because he wanted to *drop out* of medical school on the first day of classes. At our first meeting it was clear he had made up his mind to withdraw from school. He was visibly shaken. Since it was Friday, I asked him to consider over the weekend the option of staying in medical school with a reduced load (viz., taking only one major course, with some of the smaller courses). He agreed to consider this option. After our initial, brief meeting, I reviewed William's undergraduate college record. He had attained a *nearly perfect* 3.7 plus GPA (out of 4.0) at a prestigious Ivy League school and 12's to 15's on his MCATs. After several meetings in the first two weeks, William decided to continue in medical school with a reduced course load.

During these early meetings with William, which consisted of several hours of interview and discussion, he provided key pieces to the puzzle of his unexpected and unexplainable urge to flee medical school. When William began medical school, his anxiety grew in anticipation of being tested in each of his courses. This haunting image disrupted his ability to concentrate and reinforced his tendency to avoid the negative stimuli. As the semester progressed, he exhibited classic symptoms of panic disorder and more generalized anxiety related to test-taking. He would experience palpitations, excessive sweating, loss of concentration, shaking and an urge to flee during written exams. Ultimately, we recognized that these feelings were so powerful and overwhelming that they often arose in anticipation of the test-taking situation during studying for an exam, and even during the symbolic *beginning of medical school.*

During our meetings, William revealed that he did experience test-related anxiety, albeit sporadically, as far back as grammar school. Although he also experienced these feelings in high school and college, he was able to cope with them by *over-preparing* for tests. He has always been a perfectionist and he acknowledged an extreme need to please external reinforcers (e.g., teachers, parents). Pleasing these reinforcers in academic activities meant achieving 100 percent on tests. Nothing short of 100 percent would do.

As the first semester progressed, we were able to analyze the problem and institute some training in relaxation strategies. We dissected the test-taking and studying situations and identified critical events which precipitated anxiety such as *sitting down to begin studying something new* and *the first question to which I'm not sure of the answer on an exam.* The first step was to help William recognize these events and their impact, and then to provide him with strategies which helped him to overcome their initial paralyzing effect.

On more than one occasion during that first semester, a night or two before his impending exams, I would receive a telephone call at home from William, who was experiencing panic with its physical manifestations.

During these times he needed a great deal of support and reassurance. On his first major course exam he received a score of 96 percent and was quite upset because he *knew* the answers to the two questions he got wrong. During the test he experienced symptoms of panic attack (palpitations, excessive sweating) which scared him.

By the end of the semester we had made tremendous progress. William actually felt *okay* about the results of an exam on which he scored in the upper 80's because he was able to partially control his panic reaction through relaxation techniques. New challenges continue to emerge for William with each new test and new course. He is fighting to achieve control over his relationship with the medical school environment, and he is experiencing great success.

In many instances test anxiety can be ameliorated by a strong relationship with an academic advisor. Helping a student to manage severe test anxiety is often more time consuming and best accomplished by a faculty advisor working together with the student and a psychological counselor. Some students may require pharmacologic intervention as an interim or supplemental strategy. Beta blockers, for example, may be used to *jump start* progress by suppressing endorphin-induced memory loss and its anxiolytic effects.

Another affective state which is associated with a variety of learning problems is depression. There is evidence in the literature that depression is widespread among medical residents and interns (Hsu & Marshall, 1987; Garfinkel & Waring, 1981; Russell et al., 1975; Valko & Clayton, 1975; Waring, 1974). One study showed that 23 percent of house staff (30 percent of all interns) surveyed had some degree of distress or depression, which was considerably higher than the 15 percent reported in community studies (Hsu & Marshall, 1987). Few studies have examined the prevalence of psychiatric disorders in medical students. The authors of a study of psychosocial changes during the first year of medical school found that symptoms of stress (*hassles*) and depression (*negative mood*) increased (Wolf et al., 1991). Another study of medical students in Belgrade found that 16 percent had a psychiatric diagnosis (Liubomir et al., 1988). Based on these findings, one would expect that learning problems related to psychiatric disorders such as depression or psychological states such as negative mood would be fairly common. In the following case of John, we can see how such a disorder can impact upon learning and how this can go undetected in the medical school environment.

John is a student who spent four years on a roller-coaster ride through the preclinical curriculum. For the first year and a half nobody knew that he had been diagnosed previously with depression. He was afraid to share this information with anyone because of a statement in the student handbook that proclaimed students should be *physically and emotionally fit* to withstand the rigors of medical school.

During the first year he did well on some preclinical course exams and poorly on others, ending each semester with less than satisfactory performances in several courses. This erratic performance contrasted with his excellent undergraduate academic record at a highly selective college and his superb MCAT scores. At the end of this period it was decided that John should be formally tested for learning disabilities. He was administered a battery of psychoeducational tests and found to have *superior intellectual abilities* but *highly significant weakness* in memory. Concerns he shared during our academic counseling sessions validated his memory problem. He stated that he could not clearly recall facts which he studied more than a few days earlier. In addition, he had long-term memory problems as evidenced by his inability to recall names of friends and teachers. In addition to his problems with memory, he developed study problems which included problems concentrating and withdrawal; not regularly attending class. He blamed insomnia and poor sleep habits. No matter how much he tried, he could not fall asleep until 2 a.m. or 3 a.m. He felt he needed 8 to 10 hours sleep per night, thus making it virtually impossible to attend morning classes. His teachers corroborated his sleeping problem with evidence from the morning classes he *was* able to attend. They reported that he was always distracted, sleeping or eating breakfast at his seat.

Because of his memory problem he would generally wait until the last day before an exam and cram during an *all-nighter* in hopes of retaining information briefly for the exam. Through academic counseling he finally divulged that he was currently being treated for depression by his primary care physician. He felt that his memory was better without the pharmacologic treatment. Although there is no evidence that the specific medication has any effect on memory, one must consider the impact of such treatment, as well as the disease itself, on memory loss.

With intensive academic counseling, which focused on the development of memorization skills, strong encouragement for studying in peer groups, a reduced course load and the development of a fixed schedule for studying, he began to perform at the *near honors* level. However, he eventually resumed a full course load and regretfully returned to many of his former poor study habits. The task remains of finding the appropriate balance between coursework and personal growth activities which will enable him to effectively function as a medical student and physician. One might predict that he will only be able to accomplish this with an enhanced awareness of his own and his patient's weaknesses and short-comings, in an academic environment which will be supportive of his learning difficulty.

Screening for potential affective sources of learning problems is an important responsibility of faculty, advisors and administrators. If, in fact, as many as 30 percent of students experience some affective difficulty such as fear of failure which potentially inhibits academic performance, and as many as one out of ten students may be experiencing an affective disorder which jeopardizes their medical careers, then promoting understanding of these problem areas should be an important part of faculty development efforts. Figure 21 presents a series of screening questions which can be used by advisors, faculty members, or by students themselves to identify learning problems which are tied to affective sources.

1. **How well prepared did you feel for your last exam?**

2. **How well prepared do you usually feel?**

3. **On a scale of 1 - 10 (with 10 being most) how worried do you usually get about failing an exam?**

4. **How does worrying affect how you study or take a test?**
    Do you have difficulty concentrating?

5. **Are you having any difficulty sleeping? Explain**

6. **Have you felt any physical symptoms such as excessive sweating, nausea, palpitations, or dizziness while studying for, or taking an exam?**

7. **Have you ever felt the need to get up and leave during an exam just to get away? How often does this happen?**

8. **Are you easily distracted by routine things around you (e.g., people turning pages) during your studying or during an exam?**

Figure 21. Screening questions for affective problems.

Remediation of such problems will depend upon the severity of the underlying affective component. Generally, the less severe (and more common) problems may be addressed through brief counseling interventions with a faculty member or advisor. These interventions should include the establishment of a trusting relationship with the student which will allow exploration of feelings, sharing of experiences, examination of specific barriers to, and resources for, change, and the development of a plan for managing the problem. This plan will then serve as a focus for follow-up sessions with the student.

The high incidence of learning problems which can be traced to an affective source also requires that the medical school environment take measures to prevent the development and augmentation of such problems. This could include: (1) reducing stress associated with the academic work load by eliminating learning requirements of less meaningful material in each course (cf., Taylor, 1992); (2) offering a pass/fail option to reduce emphasis on competition and upon external motivation and reinforcement to achieve excellence; and (3) emphasizing formative evaluation (e.g., test-taking for purposes of identifying needs and improving knowledge) over summative evaluation (e.g., test-taking to determine if one *passes* the course). These and other suggestions for improving the learning environment in medical school are discussed in Part III of this book.

COGNITIVE SOURCE

The cognitive source of learning problems in medical students most often can be traced to difficulty in one (or a combination) of three areas: (1) written communication (viz., reading, writing), (2) spatial-perceptual ability, and (3) oral communication (e.g., interviewing skills). These problems appear with varying degrees of intensity and must be defined in relation to the context of medical school. Figure 22 presents these learning problems as continua and defines the poles at each extreme.

Most medical students who experience problems in one of these areas are only mildly affected in their learning and their performance on evaluations. There are, however, students who experience the problem more severely who may not have been identified or diagnosed prior to matriculation in medical school. Learning problems in each of these areas will be described and exemplified.

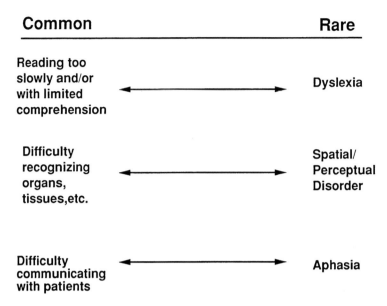

Figure 22. Continua of common cognitive sources of learning problems among medical students.

Reading

The unexpectedly widespread nature of reading problems among medical students is suggested by Guyer (1987, 1988). She found that 5 percent of students in one medical school experienced reading problems severe enough to be diagnosed as dyslexic. Developmental dyslexia is traditionally defined as above average intelligence combined with a reading comprehension score at least two years below expectation (Aaron & Phillips, 1986). It may also be defined by exclusion: a failure to acquire literacy which cannot be attributed to factors such as lack of intelligence, loss of peripheral sensory function, emotional or social problems, etc. Ellis (1985) compares developmental dyslexia to the medical model of obesity rather than to a disease model. Such a definition allows for differences in severity, accounts for the importance of environment in defining the problem, and broadens the definition of prevalence depending upon where one "sets the limit" (Aaron & Phillips, 1986). The concept of developmental dyslexia appropriately describes a small but increasingly recognizable segment of the medical student population. These students' reading problems would not easily be recognized outside of the demanding context of medical school. My experience indicates that underlying factors associated with reading problems among medical students are similar to those in the general population: (1) English as a second language; (2) low self-confidence; (3) low visual recognition and phonologic skills; (4) early educational experiences which devalued reading; and (5) absence of a reading system (cf., Ellis, 1985).

Generally, students with reading problems studied long hours in college compared to their peers. They find in medical school that there are not enough hours in the day or week to keep up with their work. Statements which are typical of medical students who are experiencing reading problems are:

> "I always have to study more than others in my class."

> "There's never enough time between tests for me to finish studying."

> "I'm always trying to catch up."

> "I have to re-read paragraphs and chapters several times to understand what they're saying."

> "I usually don't have time to go back and review my answers on a test."

Consider the case of Adam who was born in a foreign country. His father was a laborer, his mother a homemaker. Both attained a primary school education only, and mostly spoke another language at home. Adam went to a state university where he majored in a scientific discipline. His science and overall GPA was 3.4.

His first attempt at taking the MCATs yielded 8's and 9's in the sciences and 5's in both reading and quantitative. His first application to medical school was rejected. Over a period of two years, he enrolled in more college level science courses, including chemistry and biochemistry, for which he received A's and B's. His second attempt at the MCATs yielded 10's and 9's in the sciences, a 9 in reading and an 8 in quantitative. He was accepted at our medical school three years after his initial application.

During the first week of medical school, he successfully placed out of biochemistry by scoring exceptionally well on a standardized qualifying exam. Very few students accomplish this difficult academic feat (1 to 4 percent per year). However, with this reduced academic work load he failed his behavioral science course and received a marginal in genetics during his first semester (he passed anatomy and communication skills).

On average, less than 1 percent of students do not receive at least a satisfactory grade in this behavioral science course. With a full course load during the second semester, he received a satisfactory in physical diagnosis and his first year clerkship in community medicine, but failed physiology. He remediated behavioral science by an exam on which he scored a ninety-three. It was noted in his record that he would have received an *honors* grade if this was his original exam. He remediated physiology and genetics by taking them the following year.

His first semester of his third year in medical school (second preclinical year) he did not pass the second behavioral science course. He was the only student ever to fail both behavioral science courses. In addition, he failed pathology and had a *marginal* in pathophysiology. He did pass pharmacology, microbiology and excelled in geriatric medicine.

After Adam's third problematic year in the basic sciences, the academic promotion board required that he undergo cognitive testing to help explain his erratic performance. The psychometric test results demonstrated average to superior range of scores on tests of intelligence; his IQ was 120. However, marked discrepancies in his scores were highly unusual. His spelling was at the eighth grade level and his reading speed and comprehension were below the fifth percentile for his age group (ninety-five percent performed better). His overall reading and language scores were average for the ninth grade of high school.

A large part of Adam's reading problem could be traced to his poor vocabulary and inability to phonologically recognize words. Like many individuals with dyslexia, he would mistakenly associate the meaning of new or unfamiliar words with familiar words because of similarity in spelling. For example, when he and I reviewed his anatomy exam he repeated the pronunciation of the word fontanelle as *frontella* three times. The specific exam question asked about the location of the fontanelle to which he mistakenly responded *the front of the brain*. His learning process was skewed by his inability to phonologically recognize this word.

These types of word association errors combined with a very limited vocabulary (perhaps rooted in the absence of English-speaking experience at home) help explain his atypically poor performance in the behavioral science courses. In these courses the textbooks rely on advanced non-medical vocabulary skills and the volume of reading is high. Further academic counseling revealed that he had taken special reading classes through grammar school and *stayed away* from English courses in college. He had also been diagnosed with Attention Deficit Hyperactivity Disorder (ADHD).[2]

The test data and interview findings persuaded the academic promotion board to require Adam to take a leave of absence to obtain help for his reading problem. He would receive continued intensive, academic counseling and reading tutorial during this period. He would be allowed to return when he could demonstrate that he had substantially improved his reading and language ability.

Adam was re-evaluated at six months and demonstrated remarkable improvement. He raised his overall reading skills from the 46th to 80th percentile. Word recognition increased from the 54th to the 78th percentile while his comprehension rose from the 70th to the 95th percentile. His spelling score increased from the 24th to the 45th percentile. Based upon these dramatic improvements, he was re-admitted and achieved honors and near honors grades on tests in pathology and pathophysiology. He exudes great self-confidence and has been helpful in providing assistance to other students who are having academic difficulty. He continued to receive tutoring for reading and academic counseling, has since passed all preclinical requirements and successfully completed all required clinical rotations.

Adam's dyslexia is one of the more severe cases to be observed. Guyer also describes medical students with severe dyslexia and ADHD. In Adam's case, and with those students described by Guyer (1987), academic counseling and intensive tutoring in reading and study skills have enabled them to overcome their problems and satisfactorily perform the requirements of the medical school curriculum.

The most common reading problem among preclinical medical students is reading too slowly (with adequate comprehension). Typically, these students have excellent vocabularies and perform adequately on untimed exams. There is, however, for this group a large discrepancy in exam performance under timed versus untimed conditions. Often they do not completely *finish* studying for exams, feel *rushed* during exams, and make *foolish* errors because they do not have enough time to read each question carefully.

Our experience shows that an important predictor of this reading problem is a relatively low score in reading (verbal reasoning) on the MCATs. For most of these students, early recognition of the problem, combined with practicing the learning skills and strategies presented in Chapter 1, and a restructured academic environment which allows more time for selected students to complete exams, will meet their special learning needs.

Other students who experience reading problems may require more individually tailored interventions to meet their needs. For one student who was diagnosed with dyslexia, being placed in a separate room for course exams, which allowed him to read aloud each question stem and alternative, dramatically improved his test performance. This same student experienced problems with sequence, organization and accuracy in her written case histories for the physical diagnosis course. I believe that the same processing problem which inhibited reading also inhibited history-taking and presentation. Two strategies were developed and implemented to ameliorate her learning problem related to clinical performance. First, she was encouraged and helped to develop a written outline which she could use with every patient to facilitate the history-taking process. The outline included a time-line to note onset and chronology of the presenting problem, a space for a genogram to report family history, and other cues which capitalized on her *visual learning* strengths. Second, she was then encouraged to read her completed written history aloud as a check for organization and accuracy. For some students, an individualized plan tailored to meet learning needs can be implemented within the normal routine of courses. In other instances, encouraging an *extended curriculum* (e.g., three preclinical years) which will allow more study and reading time for each course may be appropriate.

Quite often, faculty members and advisors or students themselves can conduct preliminary screening which will uncover potential reading problems (see Figure 23). In the event that problems are identified, the student can consult with an *in-house* learning specialist and/or work with enlightened faculty who will personally tutor the student to improve reading skills.

Spatial Ability

Compared with other areas of cognition, precise identification of spatial abilities is a relatively recent phenomenon (Quirk et al., 1987). Spatial ability may be defined as the capacity to perceive, retain, recognize or reproduce three-dimensional objects in the correct proportions when they are rotated in space, translated, projected, sectioned, reassembled, inverted or verbally described (Rochford, 1985).

1. **How often do you immediately reread a paragraph because you didn't understand it?**

2. **Would you say that you read word-by-word, or that you focus on important words and phrases?**

3. **Do you sound out words orally when you read?**

4. **How often do you transpose letters or words when reading orally or when writing?**

5. **Do you often skip words or lines and have to 'double back'?**

6. **Do you have trouble remembering the start of the page or the paragraph by the time you get to the end?**

7. **Do you have difficulty concentrating when you read?**

Figure 23. Screening questions for identification of reading problems.

A learning problem which quite often presents during the preclinical years relates to the student's ability to examine and interpret three-dimensional images. In a recent study, Rochford (1985) found that approximately one third of medical students at the University of Cape Town begin anatomy with clearly measurable spatial deficits. He found that although most of these students acquire the necessary skills during the course without special intervention, 7 to 10 percent of all students do not acquire these skills by the end of the course. If these latter students with serious learning deficits do not compensate by excelling in non-spatial parts of the course and examinations (e.g., information-related multiple-choice questions), they could fail. My experience suggests that many students who experience this problem in one course (e.g., gross anatomy) may also experience difficulty in a later course which demands similar abilities (e.g., histology, pathology, surgery or other clinical rotations).

Research suggests that spatial perceptual problems can be remediated. There is evidence that young children can enhance spatial abilities by learning fundamentals of geometry through individualized programmed instruction (Adsett, 1968). Rochford (1985) suggests that medical students with identified spatial problems be identified and then taught and evaluated using techniques which are different than those used with students who do not have these problems.

Consider the case of John which illustrates a spatial learning problem and also raises potential ethical dilemmas for promotion boards and administrators. He came to me after his second anatomy exam because he had received a near failing grade. A review of his exam revealed that he had done very well on the multiple-choice component which emphasized factual information. On the lab practical, however, he did poorly. He exhibited great difficulty processing visual information about organs, tissues, etc., when they were viewed out of their immediate context (viz., part of the body) and cross-sections were nearly impossible for him to interpret.

During an academic counseling session, John revealed that he has extreme difficulty *seeing in three dimensions.* He said that he cannot easily distinguish between *front and back, nor right and left.* He did not have a driver's license because of this impairment. He stated that what was most difficult about driving was that he could not interpret images he observed in the rearview mirror. He also said he experienced a problem with fine motor control which was evident in the fact that he never learned to write in cursive, thus always printing his written communication, including signing his name.

Interestingly, John already had a doctoral degree (outside of the physical sciences) and his academic credentials were impeccable. He had graduated from a top college with honors.

I referred John to a neuropsychologist for a thorough diagnostic workup. This was to precede the development of an individualized learning plan which would address his learning problem and academic limitations. He met with the neuropsychologist briefly, then decided not to pursue the diagnostic workup nor further academic assistance from my office. I received a letter from John describing his decision. The following is an excerpt from this letter:

> I have decided to not pursue the testing for several reasons. First, I am convinced that the anatomy department would make absolutely no changes in how they test and do not want the department to have very personal information about me unless it would result in some change. Secondly, if the information were provided to the anatomy department, it would become part of my record. Associates of mine in the medical community strongly cautioned me about having information like that as part of my record. I do not want the information in my record because I do not want to be stigmatized as I proceed through my clinical years. Thirdly, I am doing very well in all subjects and in anatomy on the written tests. I do not want to be perceived as somehow incapable, when for most of the things I will be called upon to do, I am very capable.

> What I find most difficult about the practicals is totally irrelevant to the practice of medicine—organs disoriented, disemboweled intestines turned

upside down and backside to, etc. Clinical anatomy and anatomy oriented in the anatomical position give me no difficulty at all. So, I will suffer through the disoriented presentations, miss getting honors in anatomy because I cannot orient myself to the disorientation, and be quite content!!

I really appreciate your willingness to listen and to help me at a time when I was quite upset. It meant a lot to me. I will stop by to talk with you about the wisdom of my decision!

This case raises several issues not yet discussed in relation to learning problems. For example, what if a student who might benefit from psychoeducational testing and remediation refuses? Are the evaluation/ advising mechanisms in medical school capable of identifying all students who need assistance? To what extent should medical schools provide career counseling and guidance to students with learning problems?

Faculty, administrators, or students themselves can use the following screening questions to determine the need for further diagnostic testing in the area of spatial-perceptual learning problems.

1. **How did you do in your anatomy (cell biology) course (compared to biochemistry)?**

2. **Do you do better on the written multiple-choice part, or on the laboratory practical part, of your anatomy tests?**

3. **Have you had exceptional difficulty with geography or geometry courses?**

4. **Do you have difficulty reading maps? Following directions to a geographic location? Differentiating between left and right?**

5. **Do you have difficulty interpreting images in a rear- view mirror?**

6. **Do you prefer printing to writing in cursive?**

Figure 24. Screening questions for identification of spatial-perceptual problems.

Individual treatment for more severe spatial disability generally requires professional expertise. Thus, most faculty and advisors can play a primary screening role and refer students with these potentially difficult problems to appropriate resources within the institution. To facilitate identification of, and accommodation to, students with less intrusive spatial learning problems, faculty and administrators will need to modify the academic environment by:

1. conveying an openness toward students with spatial problems and an atmosphere of trust that will encourage students with these problems to reveal them and seek help;

2. offering redesigned educational demonstrations or a *programme of differentiated teaching* (Rochford, 1985) which address the student's deficit(s);

3. developing alternative testing procedures which rely less on slides, figures and diagrams which represent three-dimensional objects in two-dimensional space, and more on actual manipulation of objects. This is especially important while students are learning to overcome their disabilities; and

4. providing realistic and directive career counseling based upon the student's strengths and weaknesses.

Chapter 1 presents several strategies for teaching spatial perceptual skills which can be enhanced for use with students who have identified spatial learning problems.

Communication Skills

Another area of learning problems which has both affective and cognitive components involves the ability of students to orally communicate with others. These difficulties are typically identified during clinical rotations, although they may appear during preclinical courses which use role play and small group discussion to teach the medical interview.

In some instances the communication problem which is evident in the student's behavior has a strong affective component. Unrecognized feelings such as fear of harming the patient, fear of loss of control, or fear of cancer in self can relate to impaired interview performance (Smith, 1984).

In most cases the learning problem has a strong cognitive component. For example, the student may lack questioning skills which are necessary to efficiently and effectively elicit an HPI. Some researchers have concluded that the language of both the physician and the patient with the inherent differences in: (1) metaphors and symbolization of disease, (2) cultural and socioeconomic background, and (3) individual values and concerns, influence the interactional process (Simek-Downing & Quirk, 1985; Inui et al., 1982). The learning problem also may be associated with English as a second language (for the student).

Consider the case of Li, who had been receiving negative evaluations by preceptors for his inability to elicit appropriate information from the patient. He was born and educated in the Republic of China and English is his second language.

It was decided that an intensive needs assessment of Li's problem should begin with a careful analysis of his verbal behavior with patients. The best method would be videotaped, student-simulated patient interactions with accompanying review sessions. The first patient presented with a skin rash and night sweats. During the interaction the patient stated three different times that he was concerned about his *buddy*. Each time Li responded by pursuing a line of questioning that focused on the chief complaint (e.g., "Have the rashes been getting worse?"). After the interaction during videotape review with the patient, I asked Li why he didn't pursue the issue of the patient's *buddy*. At this time, the patient revealed that his buddy had been diagnosed with AIDS and was dying. Of greatest concern to the patient was the fact that he and his buddy had sex at different times with the same female partner for a period of years. Quite obviously perplexed, Li revealed that he did not know the term *buddy* and thought that the patient was repeating that he was concerned about his *body*. This provided a rationale for Li's persistence in pursuing the line of questioning about the patient's physical condition.

Li's case demonstrates that difficulty with oral expressive language can dramatically inhibit learning and also influence evaluation of clinical skills. Ideally, every student's communication skill needs should be addressed early in medical school. This would facilitate the development of individualized plans for those students who have learning difficulties which demand greater attention than the standard curriculum can offer. This can be accomplished by establishing an environment which allows monitoring of individual student performance during early courses in medical interviewing and later during clinical rotations with the goal of improving all students' ability to communicate with patients (Quirk et al., 1986, 1982). Additional programs such as those described by Stillman et al. (1989, 1990), which include the use of standardized patients, can be used to assess students' clinical skills throughout the curriculum. Implementation of such courses and programs should take place early enough in the medical school experience to develop appropriate remedial efforts for those students with identified learning problems in this area.

STRUCTURAL SOURCE

Time Management

Many college students feel that they are not effective managers of time. In one study, 75 percent of students entering a prestigious Ivy League college expressed concern about their tendencies to procrastinate (Bur Study Counsel, 1984). Research on time management among college students demonstrates its importance in relation to academic performance. Macan et al. (1990) found that students who perceived they were in control of their time were more likely to report higher evaluations of their performance, less work overload, and greater work and life satisfaction.

Studies have demonstrated that excessive volume of work is a major hurdle in the minds of preclinical medical students (Davis & Cochran, 1989; Annis, 1979; Cochran & Davis, 1987). In this regard, one study suggests that medical students are expected to cover in one day the amount of academic material which they were given two weeks to accomplish in college (Canady & Lancaster, 1985). Another study found that students devoted an average of 60 hours per week to activities related to their medical education (Spurlin, Collins-Eiland, & Dansereau, 1984), and another showed that they were expected to do much more (Taylor, 1992). This extensive time commitment due to excessive volume not only impacts negatively on students with reading problems but also upon students who have problems organizing their time.

In general, medical students who experience academic difficulty can often trace it to an inability to manage their time (Wolf et al., 1980). There is evidence that many students can improve their ability to manage time by participating in brief academic counseling or psychotherapy. One study showed that 85 percent of students with excessive anxiety related to poor organizational skills benefitted from psychotherapy which focused on the development of organizational skills (Shain, 1992).

Problems with time management do not necessarily mean that more time is needed for studying. Rather, I have found that medical students' time management problems are typically related to an inability to perform one or more of the following organizational skills: (1) prioritizing (goal setting), (2) planning (choosing the most appropriate strategies to achieve goals), and (3) decision making (adapting to unforeseen change).

In addition, as already suggested, students must feel that they are spending *adequate time* studying, though not necessarily spending the *most time* relative to their peers. In this regard, Fisher and Cotsonas (1965) found that medical school performance was not related to the quantity of study time nor to time in class.

Two important areas which often demand prioritization include: (1) physical versus social versus family versus school activities, and (2) course A versus course B versus course C. Planning involves identifying specific assignments and methods for studying during specified times each day (including weekends). Decision-making skills are necessary when plans need to be modified because of unanticipated events or lack of progress. Most students who experience these difficulties need to work with an advisor or faculty member who can help the student develop a realistic schedule and monitor its implementation.

Figure 25 presents a set of screening questions which may be used to identify students who are experiencing difficulties in managing their time.

1. **Do you plan your specific study activities before you begin each day? (e.g., which handouts you will read at what time and where)?**

2. **Do you use a written daily/weekly calendar to plan your studying?**

3. **Do you plan ahead and study in each course each day, or do you find yourself studying for one course at a time and cramming for tests?**

4. **How often do you stop studying your notes in the middle of a lecture or stop reading a handout in the middle of a section, rather than finishing before you quit?**

5. **Do you have a place where you regularly study for extended periods of time which is free from distractions?**

6. **While studying, how often do you get distracted by preparing meals/snacks, making or taking phone calls, having conversations with friends, watching television, or reading newspapers?**

Figure 25. Screening guidelines for identification of time management problems.

Consider the case of Rose. She is an exceptionally bright student with superb qualifications. She excelled on her MCATs and had a superb GPA from a highly selective liberal arts college. Rose performed extremely well by her own account when the work load was light. Compared to most students, she needed very little time to prepare for an exam. While most students need to spend four or five hours per day studying outside of class, she could spend two or three hours.

However, when the work load increased (e.g., back-to-back tests in two or more courses), she became *paralyzed* and would not know *how to start or where to begin.* As the semester progressed, she gradually studied less, averaging one hour per weekday and not at all on weekends. She would then study several hours at a time to prepare for a test.

Rose's problem organizing time was, like many other learning problems already discussed, associated with a strong fear of failure. She related the analogy of her experience as a long-distance runner. Although she would run with certain friends or alone, there was one friend with whom she refused to run because she knew she wouldn't win. In the same way, she could not pace her studying when the work load increased and the prospect of finishing diminished. During counseling she also revealed that her mother is *extremely organized and totally her opposite.*

Our first step was to identify productive time when she could study without interruption. We were able to build into her schedule one-and-one-half hours of study time in the morning before classes. She had not previously used this time for studying. In addition, she was able to regularly schedule from one to one-and-a-half hours of studying per evening. Finally, she was able to increase her morning study time on weekends (three hours each day) and to study Sunday evenings. This schedule was developed over several weeks of *trial and error.*

During this period Rose kept written records of plans (before) and results (after) for studying each day. We discussed the importance of deciding what to study and in what order, and not to worry about not studying everything. She needed a great deal of external reinforcement during this period in order to maintain her schedule. She was performing at the marginal satisfactory level before the intervention and was able to raise her grade two levels to the *near honors* level after the intervention.

In addition to enhancing the medical school environment by ensuring that students with time management problems are identified and helped early, there are several other changes which could be adopted. One study suggests that more flexible medical curricula, greater emphasis on internal motivation, and new teaching techniques which "maximize learning in the limited time available to medical students" will help students establish parameters for organizing their time in a meaningful way (Jessee & Simon, 1971).

It is clear that students who are not performing well in medical school may be experiencing problems with time management or some other aspect of structuring their experience (e.g., place of study). Faculty members, advisors and administrators should explore these structural aspects of the student's experience to reinforce and intervene when necessary.

SUMMARY

Implicit in this chapter is the concept that *adaptation* is not a unilateral process in which the student adapts to the changes and the vicissitudes of the medical school environment, but is rather a mutual process involving person-environment *fit* (Quirk et al., 1987). Over the years it is apparent that medical schools have been inflexible in failing to modify unrealistic expectations for their students. In response to such inflexibility, many students "reject the whole, taking only such parts as they find palatable" (Garrard, Lorents, & Chilgren, 1972). In the absence of such *fit* or mutual accommodation, other students, who try to achieve these unrealistic study goals, particularly those students with learning problems, may experience emotional difficulties which can be accompanied by somatic problems and include such impairments as drug or alcohol dependency. The prevalence of such problems is highlighted by McAuliffe et al. (1986), who suggest that as many as 15.7 percent of medical students could be at risk for abuse of psychoactive drugs alone. One might predict that the risk among medical students for alcohol abuse is much higher, given its easy accessibility and cost.

The experiences and research findings herein suggest that it would be beneficial for faculty and administrators in medical school to become aware of students' learning problems, feelings (such as fear of failure), and strategies of coping, including lowering their level of aspiration. It is important to acquire such a breadth and complexity of understanding, so as not to conflate this set of distinguishable disabilities, emotions, motives, and experiences under the conventional rubric of *stress*. This refinement in the frame of reference for understanding medical students' experiences is particularly important for the design and implementation of *true* curricular reforms.

Endnotes

1. Scale = Honors, Near Honors, Satisfactory, Marginal, Unsatisfactory.

2. According to the Association for the Advancement of Behavior Therapy (AABT), ADHD is "comprised of difficulties in sustaining attention, in impulse control, and in inhibiting activity level to the demands of a situation" (p. 1). Characteristics include rapid boredom, shifting from one uncompleted activity to another, loss of concentration, inability to work for long-term rewards, excessive task-irrelevant activity and excessive movement in physical tasks (p. 1).

Chapter 6

FOSTERING ENTHUSIASM
AND MOTIVATION TO LEARN

Emphasis upon individual responsibility and initiative, upon independence in decision and action, upon perfectibility of the self — all of these things serve to perpetuate more basic competency motives past childhood. (Bruner, 1971, p. 121)

To understand how to motivate our students we must first understand who they are. In the 1970s Malcolm Knowles, an American educator, adopted from the Europeans a special term which refers to adult education: *andragogy* (Knowles, 1980). The term is derived from the Greek words *ander* (stem: *andra*), meaning man, or *adult* and the word *agogus* meaning *leading* or *teaching*. The word *pedagogy,* which we typically use to refer to teaching, is derived from the Greek word *paid,* meaning *child* (Knowles, 1980).

The assumptions underlying the concepts of teaching and learning in the pedagogic model date back several centuries to the monastic *grammar* schools of Europe (Knowles, 1980). At the time, teaching was viewed as the process of transmitting to children a body of knowledge and skills which is timeless and irrefutable. This was, in fact, a period in history when most knowledge was valid for longer than a lifetime; in most instances, many lifetimes. The pedagogic model was consistent with the goal of education and the nature of the content to be taught.

It is evident that today the pedagogic model is much less appropriate for teaching, especially for teaching adults. Nowhere is it clearer than in medical education. Medical knowledge and skills are changing so rapidly that you cannot even assume that what you learn in medical school will be valid when you enter practice. In fact, perhaps as many as half of the facts students learn in basic science medical education will be outdated or invalid by the end of residency. It's quite clear that the pedagogic model of teaching, with its assumptions about how children learn and which still underlies much of medical school teaching, must be replaced by a new model which incorporates the principles and assumptions of andragogy.

The pedagogic model assumes that the learner is always dependent upon the teacher for direction and information. In many respects, the learner is viewed as the passive partner in the educational process. The new concept of teaching must incorporate a developmental perspective in which the ultimate goal is to enable the learner to become self-directed and independent in a learning activity.[1]

It is more appropriate to view the adult medical student as initially dependent upon the teacher for direction and information but ultimately capable of, and motivated by, independent learning experiences. It is incumbent upon the teacher to be flexible in the development of an educational plan and in the use of teaching behaviors depending upon the developmental needs of the learner. Teaching in medical school always should *move* the learner toward developing knowledge and skills necessary to learn the topic on his or her own. As Knowles (1975) states:

> For one thing, this implies that it is no longer realistic to define the purpose of education as transmitting what is known. . . . Thus, the main purpose of education must now be to develop the skills of inquiry. (p. 15)

Teaching to the appropriate level of learning not only enhances learning outcomes but also fosters enthusiasm and motivation to learn. This is the heart of learner-centered medical education. It is both a prerequisite to, and a result of, effective learning. Without motivation, the educational process is boring and meaningless for the learner and teacher. In instances where motivation for learning is low, learning outcomes are diminished, creativity is stifled, and apathy prevails. The unmotivated student may passively conform to the demands of the immediate academic situation even though the relationship between short-term goals (e.g., passing a biochemistry exam) and long-term goals (e.g., becoming a physician) are unclear. At the same time, despite ambivalence, this student may have to proportionally diminish the role of personal goals and involvements (e.g., spending time with a significant other or spouse). At best, this results in settling on meeting minimal requirements rather than striving to function optimally when it comes to learning. It is expressed in the all-too-common proclamation by unmotivated and disenfranchised students: "pass = M.D."

In the worst-case scenario, lack of motivation can result in excessive stress and anxiety or depression. The behavioral manifestations of such pathology can be withdrawal from school at the psychological level (e.g., failure to concentrate), at the interpersonal level (e.g. avoiding peers and teachers, not attending class) or at the physical level (e.g., dropping out of medical school or taking a leave of absence). These behaviors may be accompanied by somatic complaints or substance abuse (Quirk et al., 1987). The evidence is quite clear that motivation is an important, *perhaps the most important,* component of learning for the adult learner. It also is clear that current teaching practices in medical education often inhibit motivation to the detriment of learning and, in some instances, of the student's well-being.

One teaching strategy for increasing motivation to learn is to promote learning by discovery. We can assume that adults are goal-directed, viz., that they act in order to achieve their related short- and long-term goals. It would follow that for the learner to be motivated he/she must view the learning activity as relevant to the achievement of competence related to a long-term goal. For adult medical students, successful completion of each learning activity (e.g., learning how to elicit past medical history) can mean the progressive development of competence required to become a physician.

Teaching (and evaluating) with the goal of instilling inner directedness will not only enhance motivation but also foster lifelong learning. Learning, in and of itself, can be characterized as a potentially fulfilling and self-perpetuating activity. It must, however, be linked to one's intrinsic goals and aspirations. Upon entering medical school, learners are clearly directed toward learning to become competent physicians. Very quickly this goal becomes obfuscated by the immediate and unrelenting need to *pass* tests which assess competence in very prescribed and defined areas not necessarily *perceived* to be related to the original goal.

The loss of goal-directedness and motivation can negatively impact the learner's performance in two ways: (1) he/she fails to find intrinsic meaning in the day-to-day learning activities of medical school; and (2) the learner does not dare to take chances, viz., to go beyond what is required; to create as opposed to imitate. With respect to the latter, it is curious but true that even superior performance on tests, which is motivated solely by grades, can actually dampen the *will to learn.* In this regard, many students lose their interest in *going beyond* what is required or are deterred from taking alternate paths in their thinking. There is little interest in intellectually *challenging* teachers' perspectives (except, perhaps to have a *wrong* answer graded *right*)! Learning becomes a passive process and centers primarily on *mastering what is known,* rather than on *expanding the boundary of what is known.*

Under these circumstances, the self-prescribed goal of becoming a competent physician, with its accompanying enthusiasm and motivation to learn, is replaced by the externally imposed goal of passing exams to satisfy an extrinsic reward (and punishment) system. The long-term negative effects may include a distaste for learning which will inhibit self-initiated, lifelong, continuing medical education.

The teacher's role in promoting discovery learning is to provide the necessary skills, and a context which stimulates questions and provides the necessary resources to learners for answering them. This includes building independent study time *and* teaching students the independent learning skills described in Chapter 3.

Teaching should promote discovery. Discovering questions is as important and motivating to medical students as is discovering their answers. As already discussed, this factor is often neglected in traditional problem-based learning curricula.

In addition to promoting discovery learning, a second strategy for enhancing motivation is to encourage change (e.g., change in a point of view, methods of constructing reality). Learning can be defined as growth. As such, it represents a change from the status quo. Changing can enhance confidence in learning and can foster enthusiasm, especially for the adult learner. Suchman (1964) states: "The ability to assimilate discrepant events is intrinsically rewarding, and the construction of new conceptual models that enable one to find new meaning in old events creates in the learner a sense of power" (p. 63).

Practically speaking, change or growth is fostered by lectures and reading which expose discrepancies, inconsistencies, contrasting viewpoints, and limitations. It also includes panel presentations, co-teaching or team teaching, and small group discussion which allow for a variety of viewpoints to be expressed if they are structured appropriately. As teachers we must actively build these opportunities for change into our teaching objectives and methods.

A third strategy for enhancing motivation to learn in medical students is to minimize the risk of failure during learning. Change can be disquieting or even untenable if the associated risk of negative reinforcement of failure is too great. One of the greatest natural risks in creative learning is failure, which is viewed too negatively. Failure can be negatively reinforced to the point where it jeopardizes the well-being (e.g., emotional health, matriculation) of the individual learner and the learning self.

In many medical school curricula, the risk of failure in learning is often too great for creative learning to take place. Most often we fail, as teachers, to differentiate between failure during learning (which provides an opportunity for further learning) and failing to achieve competence *after* learning has taken place. Especially during clinical clerkships, where the window of opportunity for evaluating competence can be quite small (e.g., a student may be with a single teaching attending (physician) for only a fraction of the total learning experience), failure to learn on a *first try* is often used as *final* evaluation by that attending. It's no wonder that medical students often will not *risk* taking chances to learn if a less than perfect performance might be held against them. Stringent grading policies, combined with unrealistic learning expectations, and failure of teachers to differentiate formative from summative evaluation, enhance this risk of failure.

For the learner to be willing to change (viz., learn), he/she must be willing to take the associated risk which cannot be perceived as too great or unrealistic. Abraham Maslow (1968) provides a theoretical rationale for this view. He states:

> Every human being has *both* sets of forces [defense and growth] within him. One set clings to safety and defensiveness out of fear, tending to regress backward, hanging on to the past . . . *afraid* to take chances, *afraid* to jeopardize what he already has, *afraid* of independence, freedom and separateness. The other set of forces impels him forward toward wholeness of self and uniqueness of self, toward full functioning of all his capacities. . . . (p. 46)

Reducing the risk of failure during learning means clearly specifying and differentiating the consequences of failure during learning (e.g., feedback and practice) from final or *summative* evaluation. This will help gain the learner's trust and foster motivation to learn.

The boundaries of learning must be clearly differentiated from the boundaries of evaluation. During learning it must be perceived as being acceptable to fail. If the learner is forced to make a choice between learning (change or growth which is the natural inclination for the motivated adult) and preventing the possibility of failure which can lead to non well-being (e.g., a lower grade), he/she will choose the latter. Maslow (1972) proposes that ordinarily if there is a choice between giving up growth or giving up safety, then safety wins hands down. The medical teacher must help create a safe environment for learning in the classroom, on the wards, and in the office-based practice. Freedom to ask questions, disagree, express opinions and feelings, correct the teacher if appropriate, challenge research findings and *acceptable* answers to exam questions are all important outcomes associated with implementing this strategy.

Another strategy for increasing motivation to learn is to increase the learner's responsibility during learning. This means evaluating the importance of learning outcomes and fostering independence in achieving them. Under this condition, adults tend to focus on *real life* application of learning which, in turn, encourages self-directedness. In addition to increasing motivation, increasing the learner's responsibility for learning also should enhance retention of what was learned.

Some techniques for implementing this strategy would be to allow students in basic science courses to: (1) within broad topics, choose focal areas of study; (2) plan, develop and teach topics of interest to the class; and (3) construct parts of their own examinations. For the clinical student: (1) increase *hands-on* experience with patients (as appropriate and with full consent of both); (2) make a point to discuss routine **and** complicated cases, and *honestly* solicit student input during these discussions; and (3) collaboratively tailor a specific plan for learning and evaluating which relies to a great extent on the student for implementation. Providing guidance and acting as a resource during these educational events are important teaching activities in learner-centered medical education.

Another strategy for increasing motivation which grows out of the teacher-learner relationship is gaining the student's respect. Many of us can remember those of our teachers whom we respected as role models and mentors. This respect must be earned by the teacher. Bruner (1971) describes the process from the learner's perspective as one of identification with the teacher. The teacher becomes a competence model, one of . . .

> . . . the *on the job* heroes, the reliable ones with whom we can interact in some way. Indeed, they control a rare resource, some desired competence, but what is important is that the resource is attainable by interaction. . . . It is not so much that the teacher provides a model to *imitate*. Rather, it is that the teacher can become part of the student's internal dialogue—somebody whose respect he wants, someone whose standards he wishes to make his own. (pp. 123–4)

Teachers must strive to gain the respect of their students through demonstrated competence (cognitive side) and compassion (affective side) if they are to help motivate their students to learn. In the basic and clinical sciences, demonstrated competence lies in three areas: (1) mastery of the content of science, (2) ability to apply this knowledge or medically relevant material to medicine, and (3) teaching ability. Compassion is demonstrated in the behaviors which define the relationship between the learner and the teacher and the rules which govern this relationship (e.g., *approachability*, assigned work load, evaluation procedures). Compassion also may be reflected in the teacher's management of the relationship between the student and others, including patients.

Competent medical school faculty must highlight the relevance of the presented material to clinical medicine. In basic science courses, this must be accomplished *at every* lecture and lab. In addition to enhancing medical students' motivation, this would help faculty clarify their own teaching objectives. If you feel that the material to be presented is too *basic* or too *far removed* to spend the extra time explaining the clinical relevance, then its inclusion in the curriculum should be questioned.

In clinical rotations faculty must take the time to help students *see the forest through the trees* in difficult cases or understand the richness of apparently *simple* cases. We cannot assume that students will attain this depth of understanding simply by seeing patients or by observing preceptor-patient interactions. Students rarely have the opportunity to apply their knowledge to *real* cases in the first two years of medical school and thus need guidance in *how* to do this. Increased motivation is one outcome of such learning.

The ability to teach effectively gains respect from students who come to medical school anticipating that teaching will be *better* than it was in college (Quirk et al., 1987). Often they are disappointed. It is incumbent upon faculty to not only initially learn, and keep up with, the content of their respective scientific fields but to continually assess and develop their teaching skills. Medical schools should require teachers to participate in faculty development programs which address this important need.

Generally speaking, to enhance motivation to learn, the teacher must convey respect by *weaning* students away from dependence on the teacher in learning and evaluation to independence in these areas. Students who are taught and allowed to participate in the evaluation of their own progress as part of training for lifelong, independent learning also should be encouraged to evaluate their teachers, medical school courses, and rotations.

As part of a developmental curriculum which aims to foster independence in evaluation, faculty and fellow students should help improve the reliability of each learner's self-observations and judgments. In this connection, students could initially test themselves in a prescribed area (construct exam questions and answer them), then be tested by the instructor (or other students), and finally, with the instructor, compare the two assessments *for purposes of improving the accuracy of self-evaluation.*

Bruner (1971) helps to illustrate the importance of adult learner-centered principles in developing evaluation:

> Any regimen of correction carries the danger that the learner may become permanently dependent upon the tutor's correction. The tutor must correct the learner in a fashion that eventually makes it possible for the learner to take over the corrective function himself. Otherwise the result of instruction is to create a form of mastery that is contingent upon the perpetual presence of a teacher. (p. 53)

In this proposed curriculum, self-evaluation ultimately should be used to not only monitor performance but also to certify competence (e.g., final grade). Students would be required to achieve a sufficient level of reliability in their self-evaluations in order to continue toward independent evaluations in this *developmental* process.

It is important that the self-evaluation process replace parts of, and not simply be added to, current *external* evaluation procedures. Students quickly lose trust if they perceive these changes simply as *more work* and not in their best interest. By becoming better self-evaluators, students also will become better learners in that they will be more effective in identifying their subsequent learning needs. This is extremely important for learning beyond the *four walls* of medical school.

A final strategy for enhancing motivation to learn is to emphasize *formative* evaluation. This is evaluation which is designed solely to be *fed back* to the learner for the purpose of improving learning. It is time to diminish the heavy emphasis in many medical schools on *summative* or certifying evaluation which is reflected in rigorous exam schedules and the national exams. Students and faculty are so caught up in this externally validating, summative evaluation process that little time is left to experience the excitement of learning. Students *study for tests* every day of every week, thus leaving no time for learning from their mistakes. Formative feedback should emphasize understanding, offer constructive alternatives to erroneous thinking and reinforce positive aspects of performance. When necessary, learners should be invited to explore constructive alternatives with the teacher.

In sum, we can distill the following general guiding principles from our strategies designed to increase the motivation of medical students to learn:

1. Increase the learner's responsibility for learning. Look for opportu-

nities to expand his/her horizons, to offer new possibilities for self-directed learning. This important step will ensure *meaningfulness* and *application,* two factors which are crucial to adult learning.

Responsibility for patient care should be emphasized. Often medical students are ready for limited and *supervised* responsibility for participation in patient care well before they are offered the opportunity. For the first-year student, this can include providing patient education and life-style counseling in areas such as smoking cessation, AIDS prevention, birth control and nutrition. It can also include limited history-taking (e.g., history of present illness, past medical history, and family history) and physical exam components (e.g., blood pressure, pulse). The information obtained can be shared with a preceptor and *used* as the foundation for further interaction between the doctor and patient.

2. Increase collaboration between the teacher and learner in the planning and implementation of education. This will engage the student as a self-directed learner. From a planning perspective, find out what the student would like to learn, what he/she thinks is needed, and what he/she expects from the learning situation. Use your experience and wisdom to ensure that the student's aspirations and expectations are realistic and that the perceived needs are accurate. Although this is easier to accomplish in the one-to-one context of the clinical learner-preceptor interaction, there are ways of doing it in large groups during basic science courses. Regularly assess the students' needs and learning goals, using brief questionnaires, *real-time* classroom technologies or an interactive lecture format. The latter is an extremely important strategy to use for ensuring collaboration in large groups. Interactive lecture involves using open-ended questions to elicit students' ideas, feelings, etc., and then summarizing these experiences and incorporating them into the information base and direction of the class (see Chapter 8).

In terms of implementation in the clinical setting, take time to consult with the student before and after you see the patient. Share your information, concerns, and diagnostic impressions. Elicit the student's perspective. It is important to use the information the student has obtained from the patient if it is pertinent. If it isn't, share this perception with the student in a constructive manner. Discuss difficult cases with the student and share your past experiences. Ask the student to share her/his opinions and experiences.

3. Provide constructive feedback and positive reinforcement often during the educational experience. Elicit *corrections* from the students

themselves; encourage them to learn from their mistakes. Remove the veils of secrecy from the evaluation process and place it in a proper perspective. Evaluation should not *drive* the learning process. In addition, normalize mistakes or errors by referring to your, or other's, previous experience. All of this will encourage the adult learner to take more chances, to be creative in learning situations, which will undoubtedly result in greater learning. The safety and security associated with studying what is known to pass exams will be replaced by the satisfaction and intrigue of learning for the sake of learning. The emphasis will be on process, not content. Satisfaction derived from imitation will be overcome by the drive to learn and create new knowledge.

4. Expand the definition of teacher to include the concepts of *role model* and *resource.* As a role model, allow the medical student to know you as a real human being, not as "a faceless embodiment of a curricular requirement nor a sterile tube through which knowledge is passed from one generation to the next" (Rogers, 1969, p. 106). Offering the student a view of your *human side* which includes weaknesses, as well as strengths, interests, goals and aspirations as well as accomplishments, will gain you the respect of your students and provide them with a model for life.

Avail yourself to your students. Encourage questions inside and outside of class. Do not humiliate students who ask questions. View all questions as an opportunity for teaching and learning, not as data for evaluation.

In sum, if you treat your students like the adult learners that they are, they will reciprocate by learning more and you will have a pleasurable teaching experience. These principles of motivating the adult learner underlie the practical guidelines for teaching offered in the next two chapters.

Endnotes

1. Knowles (1980) does define the temporary status of dependent learning but does not allude to its value in a developmental sequence of learning.

Chapter 7

PLANNING AND IMPLEMENTING THE TEACHING/LEARNING EXPERIENCE: A PRESCRIPTION FOR SUCCESS

The four steps in planning and organizing teaching which are commonly recognized and used by medical educators are: (1) assessing the learner's needs; (2) defining learning objectives; (3) selecting and using at least one teaching strategy to accomplish each objective; and (4) evaluating learning outcomes. In learner-centered medical education, it is important to adapt these steps to the principles of adult learning.

It has been said that the ultimate aim of medical education is to ensure that the student becomes a self-directed learner. As such, the organization of teaching and instruction by the teacher must be viewed as a temporary or provisional state which eventually will become internalized and composed of self-directed activities. The facilitation of self-directed learning skills through modeling and more direct teaching methods is the primary goal and determines, in large part, the specific needs to be assessed and the learning objectives to be defined (see Chapter 3). We already have discussed the importance of fostering self-directedness in evaluation (Chapter 6). The ultimate goal is to foster self-directedness in relation to each step of the teaching/learning experience.

Whether it is within the context of basic or clinical science teaching, we must ensure an orderly transition from dependent to independent learning while focusing on these four steps of instruction. That is, the medical student must not only master a defined content but must also internalize the *process* of teaching which ultimately becomes the core of self-directed learning. Students must learn how to assess their own needs in a specific subject area, define appropriate learning objectives, identify the best strategies to accomplish these objectives, and select criteria for evaluating performance.

Most often medical school curricula ignores the goal of development

135

toward independent learning in students and also neglects to fully consider the educational planning process. Turning our attention to these issues will force us to reassess what is, and what is not, important for students to learn, and what really is the expected level of performance.

Needs assessment is the first step in the teaching process (and in self-directed learning). It is asking the question: What do the students (or I) need to know according to whom? Needs are typically expressed as deficits in relation to explicit goals and expectations. Formally defining learning needs means clearly establishing their importance to the ultimate goal of becoming a competent physician.

Often the needs assessment step is neglected or it is taken for granted that the teacher knows what the learner needs. The learner plays little if any role in the assessment process. From a true learner-centered perspective it is important for the teacher to formally establish and define those needs and, most importantly, to share a common perception of those needs with the learner. Not only will this potentially increase the validity of the needs assessment but also, more importantly, ensure the participation of the student in the remainder of the educational experience.

Developing a common perception may also include *accepting* the learner's perception of need. The learner's perception in large measure consists of self-understanding. Promoting self-understanding (self-assessment in relation to established criteria for success) is a key goal of needs assessment with adults and can be taught and modeled through collaborative needs assessment with the learner.

Practically speaking, in basic science courses this type of needs assessment might include the use of pretests which are self-scored by students. During the clinical years conducting a needs assessment interview at the beginning of a rotation to determine students' personal needs and objectives for a rotation is an important first step. Ideally, needs assessment data could be used in final evaluations to demonstrate change and growth.

In a collaborative needs assessment, medical students must be encouraged to assess their own levels of performance and the gap between these levels and the criteria for success. Most medical students as well as other students in higher education are disadvantaged in this regard because of their previous educational training. As Knowles (1980) states:

> Because competition for grades is such a strong element in the tradition of education, most adults enter into learning activity in a defensive frame of mind. One of their strongest impulses is to show how good they are. So the

notion of engaging in a self-diagnostic process for the purpose of revealing one's weaknesses—one's needs for additional learning—is both strange and threatening. (p. 229)

This competition is amplified in premedical and medical education, thus making the task of developing self-diagnostic skills a more difficult challenge.

The second step in teaching is to define specific educational objectives. According to one eminent educational theorist: "Educational objectives become the criteria by which materials are selected, content is outlined, instructional procedures are developed and tests and examinations are prepared" (Tyler, 1950, p. 3).

Objectives are statements, often expressed in behavioral terms, of the desired outcomes of the learning experience. The outcomes may be related to knowledge, application of knowledge and skills, or self-understanding. When defining objectives, it is extremely important to decide which level best describes the desired outcome in order to determine which learning skill(s) the student must employ. Recall that the learning skills described in Chapters 1–3 are designed to achieve objectives at each of these levels. It may be necessary to define more than one objective to cover all facets of the desired outcome. For example, perhaps learning an important piece of knowledge related to utilization will complement learning an important clinical skill in order to ensure appropriate implementation of that skill (e.g., a large cuff ensures more accurate blood pressure readings with large patients).

Well-defined objectives typically include the *criteria* by which successful accomplishment will be determined. This way the learner is clear how successful achievement will be measured. Figure 26 presents examples of educational learning objectives on different levels for medical students in preclinical and clinical rotations.

How one uses objectives to structure a learning experience is crucial to learner-centered medical education. They represent some of the believed or projected desirable outcomes but by no means should preclude deviation from the projected path in favor of creative or unanticipated learning opportunities. In fact, the teacher with the learner(s) constantly should be refining and re-defining objectives throughout a learning experience. When learner-centered medical education is properly implemented, the learners and the teacher should know that what they offer, and how they respond in the learning experience, may be used to re-direct the learning experience through modification of educational

The student will be able to...

Knowledge--Spatial Perception

...distinguish between arterial, venous and lymphatic
systems when they are located together in a section

...identify the following layers and tissues within the
vascular wall:
Tunical intima
endothelium
internal elastic lamina
valves (of veins and lymphatics)

Application--Communication

...elicit an appropriate history of present illness (hpi) in a
problem-oriented interview including:
location
chronology
quality
severity
setting & onset
modifying factors
associated symptoms

...identify and address the patient's chief concern or
hidden agenda

Self-instruction--Analyzing needs

...define his/her needs with respect to understanding
the myocardium
...identify factors (feelings) which inhibit counseling
patients about alcohol use

Figure 26. Examples of educational objectives.

objectives. This is not typically the way objectives are used after they have been distributed on the first day of a course or rotation. This flexibility, however, is a fundamental feature of learner-centered medical education.

The third step in organizing an educational experience is choosing the appropriate methods for achieving the objectives. Educational methods are the means or strategies by which one attempts to enable the learner to accomplish the objectives. Two characteristics of methods are important to remember: (1) the appropriateness of the type of method chosen is largely defined by the type of objective; and (2) methods which actively engage the learner or which result in greater learner autonomy are often most appropriate for adult learners in medical school. Figure 27 below presents a listing of the types of methods best suited for each type of objective. Each of these methods will be described below.

Level	Task	Method
I. Knowledge	Gather, encode and comprehend information	• Reading • Interactive lecture
II. Utilization	Use knowledge to gain new knowledge and solve problems	• Group discussion • Role-play with feedback • Supervised clinical apprenticeship
III. Discovery	Plan and implement self-directed learning	• Guided independent study • Practice teaching projects

Figure 27. Teaching methods related to levels of educational objectives.

The methods employed during and after the teaching encounter must be compatible with the types of the objectives defined. Generally speaking, there are three types of learner objectives: knowledge, utilization and discovery. Knowledge objectives are best met by information provided orally or in written form. Utilization objectives require that the learner be informed, and motivated, receive a demonstration, and ideally have an opportunity to practice and receive feedback. Discovery objectives, or those which involve self-assessment, self-understanding and self-initiated change, and require methods such as contract learning, allow the learner to assess, and with support address, his/her own needs which include exposing, recognizing, and challenging his or her current attitudes and feelings. Discussion during the learning experience involves allowing the learner to hear and contemplate alternative views.

The final step in effective learner-centered medical education is evaluation. Figure 28 presents the *educational loop* with all four steps from a learner-centered perspective. In the previous chapter, the importance of involving the learner in the evaluation process was highlighted. Because of its importance, and quite often its neglect, I will present an in-depth view of the evaluation process.

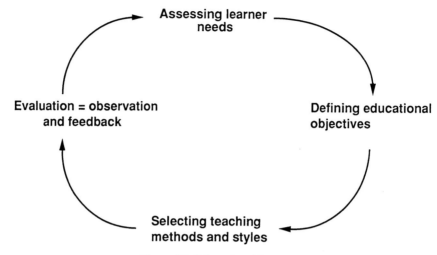

Figure 28. Educational loop.

Evaluation includes four steps. First you have to define the purpose. Second, you have to collect the data. Third, you must weigh the outcomes against the criteria for success which you previously have established (viz., objectives). Finally you must report the findings. You haven't successfully completed an evaluation until you have covered each of these steps.

There are two distinct purposes of evaluation: summative and formative. Summative evaluation is for certifying or judging competence (Bloom et al., 1971). Course exams, NBME exams and MCATs are good examples of evaluation used for this purpose. Summative evaluation directly calls into question one's competence and typically has implications for one's standing or status. Course exams determine whether or not one *passes* the course, MCATs determine *eligibility* for medical school, etc. Summative evaluation often elicits an affective response from the learner. As Bloom et al. (1971) state: "It is this act of judgment which produces so much anxiety and defensiveness in students, teachers, and curriculum makers" (p. 117). Summative evaluation is generally administered by people other than the learner (e.g., teacher, course coordinator, proctor).

Formative evaluation, on the other hand, is used solely for the purpose of improving learning (Scriven, 1967). Using *pretests* or *old* exams to identify areas of weakness and to prepare for a test, and receiving feedback based on observation of history-taking, are both good examples of formative evaluation. Formative evaluation can be implemented by the learner alone or in *collaboration* with a peer or teacher.

The second step in evaluation is to collect the information necessary to either certify performance (summative evaluation) or to improve learning (formative evaluation). In either case one needs to assess current performance. In the case of formative evaluation, one also needs to determine *why* performance doesn't meet expectations. This enhances the development of a specific plan to *improve* learning.

Performance can be assessed by *direct observation* of behavior (generally considered an objective measure) or by *self-report.* The instrument you choose to measure behavior depends on the type of behavior you are measuring. Knowledge is objectively measured using a paper and pencil test. Well-conceived multiple-choice tests (e.g., matching, one best answer) generally offer *reliable* results. What is measured is consistent from one student to the next, and the results are stable over time. However, there is danger that these tests may measure only recognition (viz., alternatives are presented) and not true recall, thus their *validity* as a measure of *useful* knowledge is limited. On the other hand, written case studies and essays may provide a better measure of recall and begin to measure use of knowledge.

Skills are best measured *objectively* using a behavior checklist to observe learner performance. This can be accomplished by a teacher, patient, peer or the learner him/herself (using videotape). There are a variety of written questionnaire scales (e.g., semantic differential) which can be used to measure attitudes and values.

Knowledge, skills and attitudes can also be measured using more *subjective,* self-report methods. The learner can report to a teacher what he/she knows, feels, or can do, *in general terms* on a written questionnaire, or verbally in an interview. In each of these instances, the learner is asked to make a judgment about his or her current level of performance.

Self-report of knowledge and behavior is time and labor efficient but often of limited value in evaluating performance. First, by nature the data is non-specific, focusing on general assessment rather than on specific knowledge and behaviors. In this regard, it offers little for either formative or summative purposes. Second, it is less reliable and valid than direct observation. Learners are going to be more or less willing and able to provide their own data. Teachers should be concerned with obtaining direct observational data on student performance of skills for both formative and summative purposes.

Self-report, on the other hand, can be used effectively in formative evaluation to determine *why* the learner did not achieve expected levels of performance. This is especially true of the adult learner who often has a mature concept of causality. He or she may be able to see multiple connected cognitive (e.g., understanding) or contextual (e.g., time) factors which inhibited effective performance. Also, the learner often has a good understanding of, and can verbalize, affective factors which may have influenced performance (e.g., anxiety). In sum, based on less than expected performance by the student on a practice exam, he or she may be able to tell us if they: (1) studied enough; (2) were confused by the lecture on protective immunizations; (3) had difficulty with the handout; (4) were anxious and upset over a disagreement with a significant other; and/or (5) didn't have sufficient background in bacteriology. With respect to identifying strategies for improving performance, you might determine *with the learner* that it would be most effective to read a selected chapter on bacteriology to improve background knowledge and then review the immunizations handout and notes with you.

Self-report also can be used to corroborate observational data and to monitor performance. Once you have established a weakness using observational data, you are less concerned with precision and more concerned with the self-perception and understanding of the learner. At this stage in the learning cycle, the speed with which feedback can be delivered is of utmost importance. Remember, the purpose of formative evaluation is to improve learning and to prepare the learner for the final evaluation. That's why it is important for the process to begin early in the learning experience and to continue throughout.

The third step in evaluation is weighing learning outcomes. At a rudimentary level, this involves comparing actual with expected performance (viz., objectives). This process, however, should be learner-centered. What is often neglected is a reassessment of expected performance levels. The question must be asked: Are the predefined objectives appropriate for this particular learner at this particular time? From a learner-centered perspective it is necessary for the teacher to be open to revising the time line for achieving expected performance levels, depending on the learner, the environment, or the relation between the two. A third-year student who has not yet taken psychiatry nor family medicine should not be expected to recognize, and effectively interview, the elderly patient with depression. In a few instances, the objectives themselves may need to be revised. For example, a physically disabled student who cannot auscultate may instead be expected to talk a physician's assistant through the procedure and to interpret the results. A student with a reading problem may not have to complete the exam in ninety minutes like the rest of the class. Ideally, changes in expected performance should be determined before the learning experience begins, but because we cannot always predict the unknown, nor the knowledge of the learner and learning situation which we will gain through experience, the teacher should be open to modifying expectations if necessary.

The final step in evaluation is to report your findings. If it is summative evaluation, the report might be final grades to the registrar, or it might be completed evaluation forms to the clerkship director. In each case the report is used to judge if the learner should receive credit and proceed to the next level of learning. Formative evaluation, on the other hand, is always reported to the learner for purposes of improving learning.

As mentioned previously, the two reporting mechanisms must be kept completely separate and this must be made explicit to the learner. In formative evaluation it is essential that the learner trust the teacher to use the data for improving learning. This will ensure openness and maximum participation by the learner. It is important to remember that the student is in a very vulnerable position during formative evaluation. He or she must acknowledge shortcomings, corroborate weaknesses and gaps in performance, and perhaps even identify weaknesses in teaching, in order to facilitate learning. If the learner suspects that this information can inhibit survival, viz., be used to determine a poor grade, then the teacher cannot expect the learner to be motivated to participate with total truth and honesty in reporting. In contrast, the learner should *not* expect that the results of summative evaluation will be fed back to him or her in the same way as formative results. Students often criticize summative evaluation procedures which do not offer opportunity for constructive feedback, despite the fact that this is not the purpose of summative evaluation.

During formative evaluation it is important, from a learner-centered perspective, that some basic rules of effective feedback be followed by the teacher to ensure behavior change. First, the teacher must emphasize positive aspects of performance as well as attempt to address the negative aspects. Students always do *some* things well and it is important to reinforce these behaviors to ensure that they will happen again. Praise is empowering and thus makes the learner more receptive to later suggestions for change. Second, teachers must learn to be constructive and not destructive in their comments. Constructive feedback not only improves learning by offering specific, positive alternatives but also helps motivate the adult learner by helping him or her begin to establish goals and objectives. Finally, it is imperative to ensure that feedback is non-judgmental and as descriptive of behavior as possible. Rather than saying that "you appear insensitive to the patients' concerns," state that "you shifted direction back to the HPI when the patient asked if it could be an ulcer."

Evidence from many sources suggests that medical students do not receive enough formative feedback. Even in clinical clerkships where the opportunity is greatest for individual feedback, one study found that 88 percent of medical students in the Northeast would like more feedback on their clinical skills (Stillman, 1989). In this context, formative evaluation sessions should be implemented on a regular basis.

In preclinical courses, one can assume with confidence that even less formative evaluation takes place because of the often very large student/teacher ratio. Collaboratively developed practice tests accompanied by teacher-learner review sessions, and small learner-centered group discussions directed toward assessing performance and using the results to improve learning, should be implemented on a regular basis. In these reviews, the teacher and learners work together to solve the problem of why the expected performance is not being achieved.

To understand the educational process as it particularly relates to *teaching in the clinical context*, it is helpful for physicians to draw an analogy to clinical medicine. The one-to-one teaching encounter may be viewed as a mirror image of the clinical encounter. Both may be viewed as interactions between a resource person (*helper*) and an individual in need (*helpee*) with the common goal of improving the latter's condition. In terms of structure, both the teacher-learner (t-l) and doctor-patient (d-p) encounters can be divided into three similar phases. The skills of the resource person are similar for both types of encounter. Figure 29 presents this comparison.

The diagnostic phase of the encounter involves a determination of the learner's or patient's needs. As such, the teacher must be a keen observer and an effective communicator. The prescriptive phase involves defining outcomes or objectives (e.g., reducing elevated lipids or being able to describe the process of RNA synthesis from a nucleic acid template) and identifying and using of methods for achieving these outcomes and objectives (prescribing a drug and exercise regimen, or reviewing a reading assignment). In this phase, expertise in planning and problem

	Step 1	Step 2	Step 3
t - l	Needs Assessment (hierarchy of needs)	Educational Plan (objectives, methods)	Evaluation (formative & summative)
d - p	Diagnosis (problem list, differential)	Treatment Plan (outcomes, management)	Follow-up (ongoing & final)

Figure 29. Similarities between the teacher-learner (t-l) and doctor-patient (d-p) encounter.

solving is essential. The final phase is evaluation or follow-up. Data may be used to certify that the patient or learner has met the objectives or to revise the prescription or educational plan. By examining each of these phases more closely, we not only come to a greater understanding of teaching but also we see how physicians can use the skills and expertise they already possess to become effective teachers.

The purpose of the diagnostic, or needs assessment phase, is to develop a common perception of what the learner or patient needs. In the physician-patient encounter it is essential that the physician can accurately and completely define the patient's signs and symptoms and understand the problem from his or her perspective. This involves sharing and negotiating perceptions until bilateral agreement is reached. The same process occurs in an effective clinical teaching encounter. The attending or preceptor must follow a line of inquiry which will lead to understanding of the learner's perspective and needs. This is accomplished using a sequence of questions which moves from open-ended to focused as more specific information is needed to characterize needs. To increase the probability that learning will take place, and to encourage future self-assessment, it is important to *verify* the perceived need with the learner.

Defining clear observable outcomes is the second step in both the physician-patient and teacher-learner encounters. In the physician-patient encounter it is essential that the physician has a clear understanding of what the patient should be able to do (bend over and touch his toes), feel (no back pain radiating to the foot), and have or be (an effective forklift operator) after the treatment has been implemented. As a result, both the patient and physician should know what to expect and be able to tell when the problem has been resolved. Clearly defined objectives are similarly an important step in the clinical teaching encounter. With a clearly defined objective (e.g., able to characterize a chief complaint including quality, location, onset, factors that aggravate and alleviate, chronology, severity as demonstrated in a simulated encounter with a standardized patient), the learner and preceptor should know what to expect and be able to determine when the objective has been met.

In both the teacher-learner and the physician-patient relationship there are generally long-term goals as well as short-term objectives. Short-term objectives should be realistic in light of the time constraints of an encounter. Linkages to long-term goals should be specified. Long-term goals should clearly be related to the learner's ultimate aim of becoming a competent physician or the patient's sense of well-being. For example, in the clinical encounter it may be realistic to think that the patient's concern about a possible brain tumor may be reduced, and that after a physical exam or lab tests completely removed; but it may take days or weeks to alleviate the actual head pain and even longer to help the patient cope with the underlying anxiety. Likewise, it is realistic to expect that a resident can define when it is appropriate to conduct a pelvic exam with a fifteen-year-old female by the end of a clinical teaching encounter, but would be unrealistic to expect that he will eliminate his discomfort with this procedure until he has practiced and shared his feelings. The latter may be one of a number of educational experiences which together would demonstrate to the resident the importance of one's feelings in the delivery of clinical care.

Methods or treatments used to achieve the goals of the encounter are also part of the treatment or educational plan. This may include methods which can be implemented outside of the encounter. Having the patient (1) read a brochure on hyperlipidemia, (2) keep a daily record of cholesterol intake, and (3) modify eating patterns by eliminating butter and ice cream are three methods of meeting the defined health care objectives. Similarly, to achieve learning objectives, a student may be required to: (1) read an article about seasonal patterns of cholesterol variations, (2) conduct two dietary assessments with patients, and (3) report the results.

The primary methods one has available within the typical clinical or teaching encounter are verbal interaction and demonstration (modeling). The preceptor or attending is limited in helping the learner achieve objectives during the clinical teaching encounter. Lack of time because a patient is waiting, meeting in a cramped hallway or office, and little or no immediate access to learning aids such as reading and demonstration materials account for these limitations. The one method which the preceptor and attending have available 100 percent of the time is their communication with the medical student.

As mentioned above, teaching methods must be compatible with the defined learner objectives. Methods employed during a clinical encounter also must be compatible with the health care objectives defined for the patient. A diuretic will reduce hypertension. A brochure will *inform* the patient who requires knowledge of the health risks of hypertension. A demonstration of how one cleans IV drug works with bleach or a role play with the patient focusing on how to convince a sex partner to *use* a condom will help the patient use knowledge to prevent HIV transmission. Counseling and the development and use of a written *and* signed contract which focuses on motivation to quit, goals, resources and barriers will be effective in helping patients to *change* behavior, quit or reduce cigarette smoking.

Finally, both the doctor-patient and teacher-learner relationships involve evaluation of outcomes for both formative and summative purposes. Patients are *followed up* and drug dosages or exercise regimens are altered depending on progress made toward health care objectives. In some instances, diagnoses are changed and new treatment methods are implemented. This same process occurs in formative evaluation of a student's progress. Extra readings are assigned, or patient experiences arranged, depending upon progress made toward learning objectives. Here, too, new needs may surface during the formative evaluation process, leading to the definition of new educational objectives and the selection of new teaching methods.

The logic inherent in the educational planning and implementation process which underlies clinical activity also underlies research (searching the literature, defining the research question, design and methods and analyses). All medical school faculty (preclinical and clinical) are very familiar with this logic yet are less systematic about its application to teaching. I hope that this chapter has provided the awareness, understanding and self-confidence necessary to encourage and enable teachers to accomplish this in a learner-centered fashion.

Chapter 8

TEACHING METHODS:
THE TEACHER-STUDENT INTERACTION

As mentioned, the teaching method which is implemented most often in medical training (as with most other training) is the verbal interaction between the teacher and learner. In this chapter, two contexts for teacher-learner interaction will be considered: (1) the one-to-one teacher-learner interaction, which is prevalent in clinical training; and (2) the lecture format, which is used often in basic science training. With regard to the former, the focus on *teaching style* might be defined as "a mode of expressing thought in language" (Webster, 1977, p. 1157). With regard to the latter, an interactive format for lecturing will be presented. Many of the ideas and principles presented for teaching in one-to-one situations and in large groups apply also to small groups. However, since there are many more variations in small group methodology, depending upon learner objectives (e.g., discussion, problem solving, role playing, etc.), it is a teaching context that requires attention beyond the scope of this book.

THE CLINICAL TEACHING ENCOUNTER

Teacher-learner communication in the one-to-one clinical teaching encounter is best understood using a system for classifying teaching behaviors into different teaching styles. The purpose of this classification system is to enable the teacher to learn the types of verbal behaviors which are best employed to meet different learner objectives.

During the past seventeen years I have presented many regional and national workshops on teaching styles. The response has been overwhelming primarily because it is grounded in concrete teaching behaviors and offers the opportunity for developing flexibility in teaching. The styles represent four points along a hypothetical continuum from the most teacher-centered (assertive) to the most student-centered (facilitative) behaviors (Figure 30). It is important to remember throughout this discussion that each of the four styles can be used in learner-centered teaching, depending upon what the educational objectives are for the student. I will address the relationship between teaching styles and learner objectives later in this section.

Assertive	Suggestive	Collaborative	Facilitative
gives direction	suggests alternatives	elicits/accepts student ideas	elicits/accepts student feelings
asks direct questions	offers opinion	explores student ideas	offers feelings
gives information	relates personal experience (model)	invites personal experience	encourages
			uses silence

Figure 30. Four teaching styles with representative behaviors of each.

One aim of the teaching styles schema is to help clinical teachers become more discriminating observers of their own teacher-student interactions. This is the first step in expanding your range of teaching behaviors so that you can effectively meet the learner's needs. The schema provides a beginning structure which you can use to differentiate among patterns of teaching behaviors. It is meant to be used strictly as a method of analyzing and improving teaching behavior and is not intended to serve as a comprehensive classification scheme suitable for use in evaluating a teacher's competence or for research on teaching. As such, its importance lies in the underlying dimension (teacher vs. student-centered) rather than in the distinctness of any one style from another.

The teaching styles schema has several advantages over other methods for improving teaching. First, it focuses attention on a minimal number of behaviors so that teachers working to add a style to their repertoire can master one aspect of that style at a time (e.g., the use of open questions), much as a beginning tennis player learns one aspect of the game (e.g., the backhand or the serve) at a time. Second, the focus on behaviors makes it easier to practice in a group context and receive effective feedback. Third, the schema's emphasis on viewing discrete behaviors in the context of a continuum which ranges from teacher to student-centered reinforces the assumption that styles represent approaches to teaching that are more or less teacher or student-centered, but that each style can be *learner-centered* depending upon the student's need. In this regard, the structure of the schema encourages the teacher to make judgments about the appropriateness of a given behavior or style only as it relates to the specific needs of the learner in the interaction. In other words, the assertive style may be used in a very learner-centered way, and the facilitative may not depending on the needs of the learner and other features of the educational context.

As represented in Figure 31, each style possesses its own characteristics in relation to teaching and learning. The assertive style includes the most teacher-centered behaviors; it is the most pedagogic style if you will. The emphasis is on the teacher's knowledge, and the teacher defines the direction of the interaction and provides information to the student. Although this style is likely overused in clinical medical education, one can use it in a very learner-centered way if the learner's need is information.

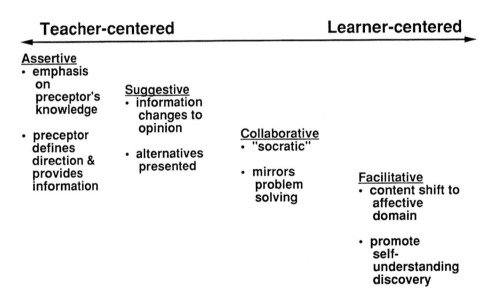

Figure 31. Characteristics of the four teaching styles.

The suggestive style includes behaviors which continue to rely heavily on teacher's knowledge and skills. However, instead of focusing on facts and directives, this style is best used when there are *options* and *alternatives* for the student to consider. By suggesting alternatives and offering opinions the teacher can help the student *recognize* and *sort through* variables and contingencies which so often result in multiple correct answers and ways of proceeding in medicine.

The collaborative style includes behaviors which are more student than teacher-centered. The character of this style is in keeping with the *socratic* method of teaching. It is the style most conducive to teaching problem-solving skills, because it actually mirrors the problem-solving process. It involves exploring ideas with the student and collaboratively thinking through a patient's problems.

Finally, the facilitative style includes the most student-centered behaviors. Because it focuses on the students' self-understanding and encourages reflection, it is most effective in teaching emotions and attitudes. When using this style, information doesn't pass directly from teacher to student.

The ability to use multiple teaching styles is a prerequisite to learner-centered teaching. The needs of the learner dictate the degree of teacher/student-centeredness, or the appropriateness of the use of each style. In this regard, the style the teacher uses must be consistent with the type of educational objective to be achieved.

The assertive style is fact-oriented and particularly suited to providing right and wrong information. It is most effective when the nature of the educational objective leaves little room for discussion. It's used best, for example, when you are teaching that there is only one correct diagnostic method to use, treatment to prescribe, or one proper way to conduct a procedure.

The suggestive style is most effective when, for example, the student needs to know the *different* courses of action available and also needs help in making a decision on which course to follow. During the interaction, alternatives are presented, pros and cons described, and the student is helped to sort through the options. Often, your opinion is offered as to the most appropriate choice.

The collaborative style incorporates teaching behaviors such as open and exploratory questions to engage the student in the problem-solving process. Using these behaviors, you encourage the student to participate with you in defining the direction and content of the interaction.

Finally, the facilitative style is most appropriate when you wish to address a student's feelings about sensitive issues. The behaviors associated with this style allow you to elicit the student's feelings and to promote self-understanding. Figure 32 presents examples of educational objectives best achieved using each style.

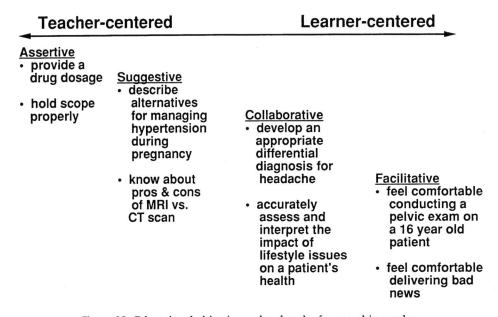

Figure 32. Educational objectives related to the four teaching styles.

In sum, the more teacher-centered styles are more conducive to teaching cognitive content and providing direction which often relates to the organic aspects of illness. The more student-centered styles, on the other hand, are more conducive to teaching process issues and affective content such as attitudes and emotions that often (though not exclusively) relate to the psychosocial aspects of illness.

There are certain assumptions about teaching styles which we can make and which have been confirmed through observation and self-report of hundreds of medical educators who have worked with the schema. These assumptions are important in helping you understand how to improve your teaching.

First, there are no *pure* interactions in which a single teaching style is used. During any teacher-learner interaction it is likely that teaching behaviors associated with all four styles will be used, depending upon the context and the educational objectives we wish to achieve.

Second, we can assume that we all have a *preferred* style which we tend to use most often. We can also infer from what we know about physicians' interactions with patients (viz., the mirror image helping relationship) that the most common preferred teaching styles are probably the more teacher-centered styles.[1] This assumption reinforces our need as teachers to become more flexible in the use of the different styles including those which are more student-centered to meet all of the students' learning needs.

Thirdly, we can assume that there are natural constraints built into the clinical teaching encounter which discourage the use of the most student-centered styles. In this regard, the collaborative and facilitative styles may take slightly longer to implement because of their interactive and often sensitive nature. However, this constraint shouldn't force us to use alternative, less appropriate styles. It may mean that we modify the teaching encounter either by extending the teacher-learner interactions or by using more than one interaction to accomplish the more student-centered objectives.

We can assume that another factor which inhibits the appropriate use of teaching styles may be the teaching style preferred by the student. We know that often students prefer learning by the more teacher-centered styles, especially if they have not experienced good teaching using the more student-centered styles. In this regard, it is easier and safer to be lead or told than to lead or tell, especially if there is perceived risk of being evaluated and failing. Sadly, this perception by students often is a reality. Thus, it is incumbent upon us as teachers to create a safe and secure context, divorced of risk of failure during learning, to encourage students to be more *accepting* of the student-centered teaching style.

In the following exercise, consider the vignettes in light of the teaching styles employed. Identify each of the teaching behaviors and the styles it represents from Figure 30 above.

Exercise:

	STUDENT		TEACHER	BEHAVIOR AND STYLE
I.	One was a slip in.	1.	Tell me about the patient you weren't scheduled to see.	_____
		2.	What do you want to talk about?	_____
		3.	Why don't you tell me about the patient you had the most difficulty with?	_____
		4.	Silence.	_____

II. He says he   1. So you've got a 72-year-old man
     feels OK.   whose only significant problem
                        during the last 15 years is
                        elevated blood sugar which was
                        controlled adequately up until a
                        month ago on a regimen of 250
                        mg a day. Now you've got it back
                        under control with 500 mg a day.   _____

                   2. When's the last time you did an
                       EKG on this man?   _____

                   3. How do *you* feel about that?   _____

                   4. What do you think his
                       problem is?   _____

III. He's not   1. I'm not sure from listening to
     dehydrating   you whether you're comfortable
     himself.   continuing him on oral agents
                       or whether you're anxious about
                       something else. Could you tell
                       me how you're feeling?   _____

                   2. What do you think is going on?   _____

                   3. But you're going to come to a
                       point where you're not going to
                       be able to control this man with
                       oral agents, aren't you?   _____

                   4. You're at a point where you have
                       to switch to insulin.   _____

THE INTERACTIVE LECTURE

A lecture [is] a process by which information is transferred from the notes of
the lecturer to the notes of the student without going through the minds of
either. (Simpson, 1972, p. 98)

The amount of thinking that takes place in a lecture depends to a great
extent upon the qualities of the lecturer and of the lecture. Flexner in his

early treatise on medical education called an effective lecturer a "textbook plus a personality" to which Simpson (1972) responds that the problem with many medical school lecturers is that "the personality may be missing" (p. 98).

There are many learner objectives which can be accomplished using the lecture format. If one's teaching goal is to provide information, then a standard didactic lecture, or a substitute method such as reading, can be used effectively. However, in most instances, the traditional lecture format should be modified to include greater interaction between students and teacher, and among students. This will provide a greater opportunity to meet objectives related to understanding (thinking) and to motivation. Conveying understanding, and enhancing affective qualities like self-efficacy and motivation, are attainable in large groups using an effective *interactive* lecturing style.

It is helpful to think of the two types of lecture, traditional and interactive, in light of Bruner's (1962) distinction between the expository and hypothetical modes of teaching. In the expository mode, the teacher develops the pace, content, and style of exposition in the presentation. The speaker alone makes all decisions regarding direction and content in the presentation while the student passively receives or listens (Bruner, 1962). This reminds us very much of the assertive teaching style.

In the hypothetical mode, the teacher collaborates with the learners in these decisions and choices among alternatives. As Bruner (1962) states: "The student is not a bench-bound listener, but is taking part in the formulation and at times may play a principal role in it" (p. 83). This mode allows the learner to participate in the act of discovery, which, as we have already discussed, engages and motivates the learner.

Interactive lecturing uses open-ended questions to elicit learners' input in making a point or solving a problem. A second requirement of the interactive lecture style as used in the context of medical school, which is consistent with adult learning, is that it must focus attention on the real-life experiences of the learners. Although all learners in a lecture may not have the opportunity to share their experiences, most learners will be able to identify with those experiences which are related by their peers.

In interactive lecturing, the group, whatever its size, assumes characteristics of, and is treated like, an individual learner in the teacher-learner interaction. The key to effective interactive lecturing is being able to shape the *persona* of this *collective learner*. The teaching process includes: (1) constantly soliciting input to assess needs and meet objectives as you would in a one-to-one interaction; (2) using summary statements to *generalize* comments made by individual students; and (3) emphasizing commonalities and consistencies among different students' comments by referring back to previous statements by, and questions from, students. By allowing as many members of the group as possible to share experiences, to receive positive feedback, to develop the direction and to have input into the content of the presentation, learners in the entire group will likely become more motivated to learn, and potentially will learn more. The teaching behaviors associated with an interactive learning style encourage identification among learners.

An essential ingredient of interactive lecturing is constructive and facilitative feedback which was identified as an essential ingredient of adult learning. This encourages learner participation and stimulates creativity and productive thinking of students in the classroom interaction. Learners must not be afraid that they will *look dumb* or be evaluated negatively if they respond atypically. In this regard, studies have demonstrated the link between constructive and facilitative teaching behaviors in class and self-initiated and creative responses in their students (Rogers, 1967).

A few guidelines will be helpful in planning and implementing interactive lectures:

1. Before the lecture, review your learner objectives and what you wish to teach with the intention of identifying opportunities for *eliciting input* from the class. Rather than *always* providing information, seek information and experiences which will serve as the foundation for learning. For example, rather than beginning a biochemistry lecture by describing the fundamental aspects of the peptide bond as it relates to protein structure, begin by asking students to describe the phenomenon. Using deductive logic as a format for teaching, their responses can then be used to review the important structural and chemical properties of amino acids, and the important aspects of size, time and energy relevant to biochemical phenomena which ultimately will be important preparation for subsequent learning of protein structure and function.

2. Don't criticize or negatively reinforce a student who does not provide information helpful in building your foundation. If it is incorrect, it is important to *gently* respond with correct information.

If the response is not particularly relevant to the topic or an opinion with which you disagree, then it is important to positively reinforce it and re-direct discussion by soliciting responses from other students until an appropriate one is elicited. These reinforcement techniques are essential in ensuring participation by all learners.

3. Be flexible and open to shifting from original objectives and moving down a different path. This may be necessitated by an unexpected expression of need by the class. For example, several students' comments might demonstrate evidence of deficiency of knowledge of chemical modifications of amino acids in newly synthesized proteins. It would then be important to shift more attention to this topic. It also is important to shift direction, if only temporarily, should new ideas or creative alternatives be presented which were not originally anticipated.

4. Finally, distill and synthesize what is offered by the class. Provide or solicit summary statements and define principles which underlie student responses. When necessary, provide supplemental information and opinion.

In sum, interactive lecture can be an effective method for helping students achieve *higher level* learner objectives. In both the classroom and one-to-one teaching context, student-centered teaching behaviors must be used to accomplish these objectives.

Endnotes

1. Byrne and Long (1978) described the predominant style of physicians they observed in more than two thousand interactions as mostly physician-centered.

Chapter 9

COACHING IN
COMPUTER–ASSISTED INSTRUCTION

In a learner-centered medical education system, the use of computers will continue to expand faster than any other method in the near future. It will become the method of choice by which the learner will access the information necessary to solve problems and perform clinical procedures (see Chapter 2 for a discussion of computer-related learning skills). As stated in the ACME–TRI Report (Swanson & Anderson, 1993):

> To practice medicine in the twenty-first century, medical students educated in the twentieth century must be given strong grounding in the use of computer technology to manage information, support patient care decisions, select treatment, and develop their abilities as lifelong learners. (p.S37)

The reasons for the expected growth in computer-assisted instruction lie in the advances being made in information technology and in the field of human learning. Computers not only hold promise as a method of accessing and managing information but also clearly are becoming a valuable method of teaching higher order thinking and reasoning. In all cases, the learner is at the center of the learning process and very little, if any, assistance or direction is required by the teacher.

One example of a program which can be used to transmit information and to train students how to access important medical information has been developed at the University of North Carolina School of Medicine (Friedman et al., 1990). It is called Inquirer and is a microbiology information data base which is designed to supplement a student's working knowledge during problem-solving activities. The data base is divided into files: the first containing "thirty-one major scientific ideas of bacteriology, such as plasmids and transduction; the second containing factual information about 61 medically important bacteria" (Bussigel, 1988, p. 15).

For purposes of retrieval, students can conduct key-word searches, such as "Find all the bacteria (in the data base) that are gram-positive rods and will cause patients to present with upper respiratory symptoms," or simply request information about a topic such as transduction (Bussigel, 1988, p. 15).

Inquirer can be used to teach students what a medical information data base is and how to access information for use in problem solving. Other programs can help teach clinical skills. For example, there is strong evidence that computer-assisted instruction is an effective technique for teaching physical exam and history-taking skills. In this connection, at the Medical College of Pennsylvania, evaluation results demonstrated that computer-assisted instruction was at least as effective as small group teaching of cardiac auscultation. The computer-assisted instruction package, HEARTLAB, developed by the Computer Science Division of Harvard Medical School (Dean, 1987) uses a sound synthesizer that reproduces a variety of heart sounds and provides graphic descriptions of physical findings (Mangione et al., 1991). At the Oregon Health Sciences University School of Medicine, TAKEHX (Take a History) was used to teach aspects of history-taking such as symptom listing, symptom characterization and symptom analysis (Nardone et al., 1987). This method of teaching proved especially effective in teaching symptom characterization.

In addition to knowledge and physical exam skills, computer programs can be used to teach the problem-solving process. Collins and Brown (1988), pioneers in the field, liken the process of learning problem solving with computers to the process of following an adult trail of experts. In this connection, it offers students the opportunity to examine their thinking, compare it with the thinking of *experts*, and to receive feedback on the steps of problem solving. This is essential to learning this process. As Collins and Brown (1988) state:

> The students' problem-solving processes—their thrashings, false starts and restarts, and partial successes—should not be left implicit. A major value in solving problems occurs when students step back and reflect on how they actually solved the problem and how the particular set of strategies they used were suboptimal and might be improved. (p. 2)

Collins and Brown (1988) use the analogy of teaching a tennis swing to teaching problem solving. A computer can replay one's swing and motion, overlaid on the expert's, and highlight the crucial features to attend to (e.g., leg, shoulder positions). This process can be captured in time using graphic representation. The same could be done with the crucial features of problem solving. With this type of *abstracted replay* and *spatial reedification* using computation, the student is able to focus on critical features of both the self and the expert (Collins & Brown, 1988).

At the University Hospital of Leiden, Verbeek (1987) has developed and refined a program which teaches medical problem solving. It focuses on the three phases: data collection, diagnosis and treatment. A difficulty, however, is that students are presented with questions to ask rather than required to generate them spontaneously. Although students are presented with both relevant and irrelevant questions from which to choose, this type of program can only teach problem solving based upon recognition, a true limitation.

There is evidence that computer application can be an effective method of learning diagnostic skills without relying on recognition. This is the most helpful when there is standardization of descriptions of patient findings and disease signs and symptoms (Bishop, 1985). As computer programs become more adept at handling complex characteristics of the *real* diagnostic context such as probability, interactional effects of concurrent diseases and developmental stages on variants of disease, they will become more effective methods of teaching clinical problem solving. One example of such a program is a decision support tool which provides graphic displays of test values by disease states and probabilities of occurrence (Lyon et al., 1991).

Like any good coach, the role of the teacher should be to prepare the learner for the interaction between learner and computer, by developing skills and modeling expected behavior. During the learning experience or match, the teacher/coach should provide support and motivation and help the student diagnose and solve problems that arise. This is especially important in the early stages of computer-assisted instruction. Ultimately, however, the goal should be to enable the learner to interact independently with the computer to accomplish learning tasks. These tasks may involve information management, clinical problem solving or any number of independent learning activities. As Collins and Brown (1988) state:

> We need to create environments where students can flounder and where the system helps students profit from this floundering by making it explicit and, if necessary, by having coaching systems highlight the floundering and help students discover or understand better metacognitive strategies grounded on their particular experience. (p. 9)

Ultimately, the benefit of computer-assisted instruction is not that it necessarily teaches better than teachers but rather that it can complement teaching by teachers and *assist* students in a self-directed learning format (Lyon et al., 1991). That is, the most important outcome improvements when comparing computer-assisted instruction with traditional teaching should be measured in terms of students' utilization of *independent learning* skills and the enhancement of attitudes that facilitate adult learning such as motivation, efficiency, and independence.

Computer-assisted instruction can be an extremely useful teaching method in a learner-centered approach to medical education. First, it is interactive teaching which is directed to the specific needs of the learner. In the case of information retrieval it is the learner who initiates and defines the search. In the case of problem-solving learning, the student chooses a course of action based on feedback from the computer. Second, it is the learner him or herself who participates directly in the definition of learning needs. In the teaching-learning process the student functions as an independent learner and the computer as a resource. Third, it is designed to teach learning skills as well as provide information. The act of learning to use computer hardware and software is the act of developing independent learning skills which ultimately will enable further learning. Finally, it is the learner who directs the learning exercise based upon feedback generated through the interaction thus providing a mechanism for self-evaluation and responsibility for learning. As we have seen, self-evaluation, using information from multiple sources, is a cornerstone of learner-centered education.

It's clear that with these advances in teaching technology there is great potential for learner-centered medical teaching. Once students have participated in effective computer-assisted instruction activities and no longer need the assistance of coaches, they become the teachers and teaching becomes learning.

SUMMARY OF PART II

The goal of teaching should be to advance learning skills as well as to enhance a body of knowledge. Learning skills should be developed and reinforced at the same time that medical content and skills are taught. With respect to the latter, for example, when the goal is to provide scientific information, the teacher should ensure that the information is well organized, amendable to establishing meaning, and provided in a timely fashion to enhance reading and memory. In addition, the strategies necessary for this learning (e.g., organizing) should be illustrated, modeled and taught.

Teaching should promote and support independence, rather than dependence, activity rather than passivity, and relevance in learning. Teachers should be flexible in the use of behaviors to accomplish these goals. For example, in the one-to-one context, teachers should master the use of different teaching styles. When groups of learners are involved (e.g., lecture), teachers should facilitate interaction. In settings where students can learn independently, teachers should coach them using computers. Even when the primary objective is to impart knowledge, there should be provisions for the adult learner to supplement information provided using one method (e.g., lecture) with knowledge provided using another (e.g., reading, computerized data base).

Finally, teaching in all settings must be systematically planned, organized and implemented following steps similar to those followed in the physician-patient encounter (and in research, for that matter). Teaching must be viewed as a series of planned and systematic behaviors which are used to accomplish the goal of learning.

Part III

THE MEDICAL SCHOOL ENVIRONMENT

I n this book so far we have considered learner-centered medical education from the perspectives of the learner and of the teacher. To effect
meaningful change and growth toward learner-centeredness it is imperative that we also consider the medical school environment in which
learners and teachers act. For our purposes, the medical school environment can be viewed from both an organizational and a curricular
perspective. The former includes the institutional aims, and structure,
and the roles of all participants, while the latter includes specific content
and the manner in which it is presented.

The term organization is often used to describe the structural and
procedural aspects of an environment. It refers to how the various parts
are combined to constitute the whole and to the variety of roles that
people in the environment adopt to ensure that institutional aims are
achieved. The educational organization can have a significant impact on
the actual teaching-learning process. As Knowles (1980) states: " . . . an
organization is not simply an instrumentality for providing organized
learning activities to adults; it also provides an environment that either
facilitates or inhibits learning" (p. 66). Learner-centered medical education requires an organizational climate which places the learner and
learning first. This is very difficult to achieve in a setting where service
and research vie with education for attention.

In this section, I will examine the commitment of medical schools to
the educational mission and to the personal growth of its members. This
includes emphasis on fostering physical, emotional, interpersonal and
sociocultural as well as cognitive development of the learners and teachers.
It is also reflected in the recognition and facilitation of *critical transitions*
or developmental milestones in the relationship between the learner
and the environment.

I also will consider the structure of the medical school curriculum, which is most broadly defined as a collection of formal and informal teaching/learning activities typically grouped into courses and clerkships. I will examine the implications of learner-centeredness for curriculum development and implementation and offer some suggestions.

Chapter 10

ESTABLISHING A LEARNER-CENTERED CLIMATE

Attending medical school constitutes an extraordinarily large portion of a medical student's world. Typically, the related learning activities occupy the majority of hours in a student's life. He/she is expected to actively engage in lectures, small group discussions, labs, or individual learning experiences such as preceptorships and clerkships.

The course schedules are often the product of many hours of work and deliberation by faculty and administrators. These schedules include time for course work, examinations, study, and leisure.

There are implicit and explicit rules and regulations that govern the use of amphitheaters, study carrels, computers, copy machines, labs and lab equipment, old exams, recreational facilities, soda machines, etc. Students may or may not have input into developing and enforcing the rules that govern each of these activities.

Like other educational organizations, medical students are expected to continue their learning activities outside of the formal boundaries of the classroom. This consists primarily of several hours of studying per week but also could include participation in voluntary preceptorships, attending faculty rounds and conferences or volunteering in the community.

In short, the organizational features of the medical school are little different than those of other organizations except that the student members are more immersed in its activity than is typical of most educational or occupational organizations. This immersion has implications for the development and well-being of the learner.

Describing medical school in this manner accentuates the need to foster self-esteem, self-expression, motivation, comfort, and trust in the learner and teacher. These attributes are especially important for learning to take place in this environment. Medical schools must be committed to fostering them if they are to be successful in achieving learner-centered medical education. As Knowles (1980) states:

No educational institution teaches just through its courses, workshops, and institutes. . . . They all teach by everything they do, and often they teach opposite lessons in their organizational operation from what they teach in their educational program. With this deepened insight that it is the total environment that educates, we are having to rethink the meaning of an organization as an environment for learning. (p. 67)

It is essential to recognize and to develop specific features of the medical school environment which shape the learner and teacher, affectively, valuatively, culturally, ethically, and interpersonally as well as cognitively. In this chapter I will identify these important features of the environment common to most medical schools and provide guidelines for enhancing their learner-centeredness.

TEACHERS

In Chapter 7, the benefits of using formative evaluation for learning were described. Similarly, an organizational structure which continuously provides positive and constructive feedback to all of its constituents will enhance their motivation to conduct the day-to-day teaching and learning activities. To enhance self-esteem and motivation, as well as to improve teaching, faculty should be rewarded for successfully developing and implementing course and other curricular innovations. The academic benefits to the teacher of engaging in successful teaching should be as great as the benefits accrued from publishing in journals or receiving research grants.

Rewards for teaching should include positive feedback offered directly and personally from those in the administration who are integrally tied to the educational process such as chairs and deans. Professional recognition in the form of promotion and, if applicable, tenure should be offered. Additionally, it should include financial reward in the form of salary compensation *from the organization* for the percentage of effort directed to teaching. The value of this compensation should be on a par with the research funding provided by external agencies.

Such recognition for teaching should be the result of an internal peer review process developed by the faculty with the administration. A standing *committee on teaching* composed of faculty with special stature in teaching who are elected by the faculty at large should establish the criteria and be responsible for implementation and oversight of the reward and incentive program. These committee members similarly would receive financial support and recognition from the institution for participating. Just as those who excel in research receive external funding as a reward, so too should those who excel in teaching be rewarded. Such a reward system would enhance motivation and self-confidence of teachers and, from an organizational perspective, help ensure that more time and energy is devoted to good teaching.

Development and implementation of such a program will be difficult. On the one hand, there is intense pressure within medical schools for the administration to compensate for decreases in external research funding. On the other hand, this decreasing pool of money forces faculty to spend greater time and effort competing for research funds or clinical dollars rather than engaging in teaching. Such pressures on the organization must be recognized, and their negative impact upon teaching (and ultimately learning) must be averted.

An aspect of reward which can have a dramatic impact on faculty commitment is the importance of teaching relative to clinical service and research in deciding faculty personnel actions. In most medical schools, research and service are still considered more important than teaching as criteria for promotion and tenure. As such, faculty members' motivation to teach diminishes in light of the pressure to do research or see patients in order to achieve career goals. Faculty who are interested in teaching more, and in learning how to teach more effectively, do not typically receive the faculty status they deserve.

If we are to preserve and enhance the quality of medical teaching by fostering the motivation of our faculty to teach, then these organizational incentives are absolutely necessary. The movement toward learner-centered teaching described in this book inevitably will require extra effort by faculty. If the organizational structure doesn't support this movement by rewarding teachers for teaching, then there is no chance that the suggested innovations will be adopted. A call for learner-centered teaching must be accompanied by a teacher-centered organizational policy of recognition and reward if it is to be heard. This is accomplished by maintaining a climate of growth and development for faculty within the medical school.

In addition to being rewarded for their teaching efforts, faculty should feel that they are integral members of the organization. To enhance self-expression and trust, they must share in the administrative decisions which affect their well-being. Faculty should have significant representation in the development and implementation of organizational activities which affect their academic roles and positions. For example, it is essential that faculty actively participate in the budgetary operation of the medical school. In this connection, a standing faculty budget oversight committee, which has access to all necessary budgetary information, can advise the administration on important financial matters which impact on teaching such as new program development as well as retrenchment and program cuts due to financial exigency. In a similar fashion, faculty also should be responsible for developing and implementing educational policy, student affairs and student admissions. Faculty who assume these administrative responsibilities should be rewarded appropriately.

Other important matters concerning the operation of the medical school and its faculty which typically are managed by the administration, such as expansion, definition and change in mission, and defining its relationship with other health care organizations in the community, should include substantial, if not equal, representation in decision making of faculty.

LEARNERS

In the creation of a climate which enhances motivation and promotes self-directed learning, it is essential that students have significant representation on important decision-making committees that will determine their educational experiences and their lives. This includes curriculum committees, faculty personnel action committees, student affairs committees, educational policy committees, student evaluation boards, etc.

Significant representation means more than one or two students who are selected to attend committee meetings. Often these few students are expected to represent the entire student body. Instead, it means that a substantial and *representative* number of students who are elected by their peers will play a significant role in shaping the educational experience of all learners.

They will help establish and implement rules and regulations and help determine the nature of their educational experiences. They will hold offices on these committees and maintain a significant voting authority. They will receive academic credit for their participation and it will be duly noted in their academic records. This collaboration among learners, teachers, and administrators will empower learners by allowing them to share control of their own educational experiences.

Involving learners in the governance of the organization will enhance motivation to learn, foster maturity and create a climate of trust. As students assume greater responsibility, they learn to trust faculty and administrators. Also, the latter will learn to trust that students can help make sound decisions concerning their educational experience. An additional benefit will be that faculty and administrators will be required to clarify and sharpen their assumptions about teaching, learning and curricular content.

This view of organization is based upon a democratic philosophy which underpins relationships among adults and lies at the foundation of a mature society. As Knowles (1980) states:

> A democratic philosophy is characterized by a concern for the development of persons, a deep conviction as to the worth of every individual, and faith that people will make the right decisions for themselves if given the necessary information and support. It gives precedence to the growth of *people* over the accomplishment of *things* when these two values are in conflict. It emphasizes the release of human potential over the control of human behavior. In a truly democratic organization there is a spirit of mutual trust, an openness of communications, a general attitude of helpfulness and cooperation, and a willingness to accept responsibility, in contrast to paternalism, regimentation, restriction of information, suspicion, and enforced dependency on authority. (p. 67)

Implementing these recommendations would enhance respect for the organization. Medical schools must be perceived as real: with strengths and weaknesses, clear goals and aspirations, yet constantly developing to meet new needs. They must not be afraid to take chances, to grow, to change their minds when necessary, admit their shortcomings and forge ahead when there is a better way to proceed. These characteristics which we expect of our students, and want our faculty to model, should be exemplified in our organizational structure. As Knowles (1980) states:

> So if its purpose is to encourage its personnel, members, or constituents to engage in a process of continuous change and growth, it is likely to succeed to the extent that it models the role of organizational change and growth. This proposition suggests, therefore, that an organization must be innovative as well as democratic if it is to provide an environment conducive to learning. (p. 67)

I am not suggesting that a medical school organization devalue tradition and not be cautious and thorough in making changes. On the contrary, for meaningful and lasting change to take place, tradition must anticipate restraint and caution should prevent change for change sake.

One way in which the value for tradition is reflected in an organization is in its cultural competence or its ability to serve all of its constituents. This is the ability of the medical school administration to recognize diversity (age, gender, ethnic, etc.) which characterizes our culture and promote it in the areas of student admissions, curriculum and student affairs. It is precisely in this area where tradition and growth intersect. It is important that medical schools view themselves as harbingers of growth, on the frontiers of society, education, and health care reform. It is the future, with a healthy respect for the past, that orients their growth. It is flexibility and responsiveness to the needs of learners which characterize this climate of growth.

LEARNER–ENVIRONMENT RELATIONS

Another feature of a learner-centered climate is attention paid to the developing relationship between the learner and the environment. This is based upon the assumption that everyone is inextricably bound to their environment and must adapt to changing conditions in this relationship. Important events which define this relationship between persons and their environments include the critical transitions they experience along the way.

Two important transitions for learners in medical school are: (1) from college, graduate school, or work into medical school and (2) from preclinical to clinical training. Because the transitions into medical school and into the clinical years involve a major re-orientation of skills, values, roles, etc., for many students, they can, if not purposefully planned for and facilitated, lead to less than optimal functioning for students on many levels. There is a great deal of current evidence which suggests that medical schools are not adequately attending to these transitions.

At the physical level, for example, there is evidence that during these important transitions, a significant number of students experience somatic equivalents of emotional conflicts such as fatigue, headaches, eating disorders, etc. (Quirk et al., 1987; Thomas, 1976). Adsett (1968) found that first-year medical students averaged about four annual visits to the student health center for such physical complaints. Other studies have found that some students experience psychological dysfunction such as increased anxiety, decreased self-esteem, and depression (Quirk et al., 1987; McMurray, Fitzgerald, & Bean, 1980). These physical and psychological problems sometimes can lead to, or combine with, alcohol or drug abuse (Phifferling, Blum & Wood, 1981; McAuliffe et al., 1986).

During the transition into medical school, many students find that the heavy academic requirements interfere with, or alter their relationships with, other people (Quirk et al., 1987). Since the academic demands of medical school are so imposing, time once spent with significant others now must be sacrificed for studying. Students are often forced to redefine their priorities and re-arrange short- and long-term goals. This is extremely difficult to do without the support of others who are familiar with the problem and can offer possible solutions. If accomplished thoughtfully and with the support of others in the organization, resolution of such problems can be extremely growth-enhancing. Establishment of strong mentoring and counseling systems, support groups, and *open door* policy with the administration will help learners clarify values, work out compromises, and learn to communicate effectively with others about emotional issues. An organization which attends to the valuative and affective needs of its learners during transitions will produce better learners and physicians.

A specific transition event for the new medical student which offers the opportunity for personal growth is the introduction of the cadaver. The cadaver is an excellent method for teaching about the anatomical features of the human body. It also offers the opportunity to teach about many issues pertaining to the values and emotions of the medical student. For example, this brings to the forefront the personal issue of death and dying. A learner-centered organization which is responsive to emotional and valuative needs of the learner would ensure opportunities for personal growth in this area.

Similar opportunities for the organization to promote valuative and affective growth of its learners occur during the transition into clinical years. When confronted for the first time with *real* patients for whom they are responsible, new clinical students often feel helpless, incompetent, insecure, or guilty that they don't remember everything from the basic sciences (Quirk et al., 1987). These feelings can trigger or exacerbate generalized anxiety or, in rare cases, lead to withdrawal from medical school or depression. Students should prepare for this transition by learning about what to expect, *normalizing* their feelings and experiences, and developing skills and coping strategies which will facilitate the process.

During transitions, adaptation is not a unilateral process in which the student one-sidedly accommodates to the changes and the vicissitudes of the medical school environment, but rather should be viewed as a mutual process involving person-environment *fit* (Stokols, 1978; Wapner,

1987). Medical schools should help to ease the transitions by changing those aspects of the curricular and extracurricular environment which put undue pressure on students with little or no benefit to learning. In addition to new teaching and testing strategies, faculty and course coordinators should be trained in students' expectations, academic and non-academic goals, and feelings related to transition. They should become sensitive to *where* students are in the transition process "so as not to conflate this set of distinguishable emotions, motives, and experiences under the conventional rubric of *stress*" (Quirk et al., 1987).

In an organizational climate which is conducive to growth it is expected that faculty will be on the lookout for, and be able to recognize, students who are experiencing *difficult* transitions. They should know how to deal with these students and have the resources (including time) to be facilitative mentors.

The curriculum should provide opportunities for students to formally or informally discuss difficulties of transition in support groups during and outside of courses. In addition, there should be flexibility to tailor the curriculum to meet student's special needs during critical transitions without fear of reprisal or discrimination (e.g., extending one's curriculum to balance medical school with a spouse's career). In addition, the organization should provide educational resources, such as a strong counseling center and an effective screening and referral system, to help students make it through the critical transitions which all students experience (e.g., into the first year), as well as those unique to each student's experience (e.g., breaking off a relationship with a significant other, having a child). Understanding and addressing medical students' experiences and needs in light of their person-environment relationships is particularly important for medical schools as they engage in the design and implementation of curricular reform.

Chapter 11

REVITALIZING THE CURRICULUM

Curricular reform has long been a popular call to arms in medical education. In 1925, Abraham Flexner strengthened the image of medicine as science in his book entitled: *Medical Education.* He stated:

> On the ground of the increasingly successful effort to expel superstition, speculation, and uncritical empiricism from medicine, and to base both knowledge and practice on observation, experiment and induction, the present volume discusses the science of medicine. (1925, p. 4)

Since Flexner's time, and in many respects as a result of his writing, a great deal of planning has gone into medical school curricula. The predominant model for medical school curriculum today embraces the duality of medical training suggested by Flexner: preclinical training in basic sciences with a foundation in experimental research, and clinical training in the specialties with a focus on diagnosis and treatment.

Flexner's proposed structure for medical education ultimately would increase the integrity of medicine by addressing the low standards and poorly organized curricula of the late 1800s and early 1900s. This call for change was consistent with the directives of the American Medical Association (AMA), Association of American Medical Colleges (AAMC), the newly created National Board of Medical Examiners (NBME), and the leaders of implementation like Johns Hopkins. It is ironic that this curriculum reform movement which was led by Flexner (1925) has resulted in the modern practice of medical education with overbearing emphasis on scientific content despite his original disclaimers that: (1) he "does not mean that practitioners should all be experimenters or that investigators must all be practitioners" (p. 12); and (2) that the essential basic science facts "must be acquired, not as inert knowledge, but as themselves exemplifications of scientific procedure" (p. 13).

In his report to the overseers, President Derek Bok (1984) of Harvard painted a gloomy picture of contemporary medical education. He provided a compelling argument in favor of once again modifying the medical school curriculum. He alluded to the problems that students experience with the often overwhelming amount, and sometimes irrelevant nature, of material to be learned in the first two years. He also decried the often passive roles they must play on the wards in the clinical years. He disappointedly acknowledged that these problems, which are largely created by the medical school curriculum, not only diminish learning, but can result in student impairments ranging from stress to cheating and even dishonesty with patients. Bok (1984) implies that teacher-centered medical education wastes valuable learner time:

> . . . there is good reason to look for ways to improve the present situation, for the time given to medical training takes up years of human life, years that have value quite apart from whether a better doctor emerges at the end. (p. 39)

The source of the problem according to Bok and contemporary medical educators (cf., Inui et al., 1992) lies in the structure of medical school curricula. It begins with premedical education in college and continues throughout preclinical and clinical training. Many of the specific problems involving the content which is taught, and how it is taught and learned, have been addressed in the two previous sections of this book. However, most if not all of the proposed solutions to these problems would be difficult to implement without a curriculum which is conducive to learner-centered medical education.

How should a learner-centered curriculum be structured? What are the goals of a learner-centered curriculum? Both of these major questions will be addressed in this chapter.

STRUCTURE OF THE CURRICULUM

Nearly three quarters of the top administrators of medical schools agree that reform of the current system is necessary (Cantor et al., 1991). The symptoms of *dis-ease* in medical school organizations are: (1) the ever-expanding curricular content, which is precluding potential applicants from considering entering the profession because of the length of training, and preventing otherwise capable students from finishing because of the work load; (2) the ever-increasing cost of tuition, which has risen substantially over the last 30 years from about $1,000 per pupil in 1960 to over $18,000 in 1993 in private medical schools (Petersdorf, 1991); and (3) the myriad of personal problems related to learning that students face ranging from lowered aspirations to emotional, intellectual and physical burnout. These symptoms must be addressed by not only adopting learner-centered teaching and learning strategies but also by reforming the structure of the medical school curriculum.

Structure refers to the parts and how they are configured to constitute the whole. To accomplish an effective structural analysis of the symptoms one must assess the curriculum on a macro and a micro level. On a macro level, we can examine the relationships among premedical, preclinical, clinical and residency training components. On a micro level we can examine how courses and rotations are put together and taught. Important features of a structural analysis include issues of time (allotments, sequencing), roles of faculty and learners, relationships (e.g., among the faculty and administration), and functional features (e.g., cost). I will begin by considering the *big picture* and work my way down to the smallest parts.

In the *preclinical* experience students not only spend too much of their time trying to ingest new information, they often rehash the same information they learned in college or graduate school. This is especially disappointing for these adult learners who are yearning for learning experiences which involve application of knowledge and which involve responsibility.

Much of the material already learned in pre-medical curricula is repeated in its entirety in medical school in a more compact format. This may be inferred from the data that indicate that 45 percent of applicants to medical schools majored in biological sciences and another 20 percent in the physical sciences (AAMC, 1992). Repetition is not only evident in applicants' majors but also in the courses they took. A study at UCLA School of Medicine found that "the vast majority of the [medical] student's college courses had been in the natural sciences" and that 77 percent of the basic and clinical science faculty felt that this is the way it should be (Doblin & Korenman, 1992). In that study the authors found that two thirds of the medical students' course work in college had been in the natural sciences. This is not only sanctioned but reinforced by medical school admissions committees which look very favorably at candidates with such academic experience. For example, the AAMC requirements catalogue (AAMC, 1992) lists some medical schools which require or *encourage* applicants to take biochemistry, despite its own warning that:

> The practice of taking additional science courses that cover material taught within the medical school curriculum in the belief that they will be useful in

gaining admission to and succeeding in medical school should not be recommended. (p. 18)

In addition, of the 1,741 applicants to the 1991–92 entering class who *majored* in biochemistry, 61 percent were accepted (AAMC, 1992). Many other applicants who were accepted majored in microbiology, physiology and zoology.

One approach to dealing with this problem of repetition is to reduce the amount of time for premedical requirements in college. It has often been noted that medical school applicants lack breadth of training in the social sciences and the humanities. Reducing natural science requirements and increasing requirements in these other disciplines in premedical curricula is advocated by many educators (e.g., Bok, 1984; Thomas, 1983).

Despite its logic and appeal, this approach has not worked for several reasons. First, medical school admissions committees still look first and foremost at science GPA and the number of science courses. Second, students who either are primarily interested in advanced study in the sciences or those who want a competitive advantage (in admissions or matriculation) will continue to take medically oriented science courses in college. Third, many colleges are interested in demonstrating significant placement of graduates in medical school and thus are likely to give medical school admissions committees what they want.

Limiting college students' exposure to advanced natural and physical science studies related to medicine also may have disadvantages. This action might preclude college students from gaining an accurate and early *feel* for their abilities and interests in this area. Waiting until matriculation in medical school to encourage students to fully *test the waters* in science could be a disservice to both the learner and to medical schools.

A second approach to the problem of overload and redundance is to reduce curriculum content and overlap in medical school by eliminating medical school courses which can be (and often are) taken in college. Standardizing pre-medical requirements combined with a reduction of the well-recognized overlap between the fourth year of medical school and the first year of medical residency could result in a three-year medical school curriculum leading to the M.D. degree (specialization and residency training to follow).

In order to accomplish this, college students interested in medicine would take *foundation courses* which include the essential elements of biochemistry, cell biology, microbiology, genetics, psychology (normal and abnormal development), ethics, and physiology in their third and fourth year of college. Many premed students already take these courses (or substantial portions of them) in college and, as we have noted, even major in these areas. Often they use the same textbooks they will see again in medical school. Students who decide late to go into medicine could, as they do now, take graduate courses in these subjects prior to matriculation. In all instances, applicants would have to demonstrate proficiency in these areas on standardized tests *before* they enter medical school.

Such an effort to revise the overall structure of medical education would demand close collaboration and coordination of effort among faculty and administrators from colleges, medical schools and the AAMC. Considering the duplication and insignificance of some science content at both the premedical and preclinical levels, it is conceivable that the entire science *foundation* could be presented in two one-year-long undergraduate college courses as recommended for premedical training by the faculty at Harvard (Bok, 1984).

A standardized premedical curriculum also should include foundation courses in human behavioral sciences. As recently as 1991, data indicate that only about ten percent of medical school applicants majored in social science or the humanities (AAMC, 1990). Only thirteen percent of the 1991–92 entering class majored in any non-science subject (AAMC, 1992).

Requiring undergraduate courses in behavioral science and ethics in a new premedical *foundations* curriculum would actually broaden the liberal arts background of most medical school applicants and achieve the goal of breadth of training. In 1993, only 17 of 117 medical schools required applicants to have a course in behavioral and/or social sciences (AAMC, 1992). Under the current structure most medical students certainly are not receiving adequate training in behavioral and social sciences. In 1991, less than 20 of the 127 medical schools required undergraduate courses in humanities and social sciences (Ashikawa, 1991). Adding these requirements in a standardized premedical curriculum would satisfy the proponents of greater representation of humanistic and behavioral training in those admitted to medical school (Thomas, 1976).

If these *foundation courses* are required and taught in premedical curricula, *basic and behavioral* scientists in medical schools could focus their attention on the *application of knowledge* to clinical problem solving and creative thinking. The first year and a half of medical school would be able to focus on these problem-oriented, *application* learning experiences for students. To support the learning process in medical school and beyond, another longitudinal course would focus on all the learning skills necessary to learn medicine.

The preclinical curriculum should include problem-based learning courses which are team taught by basic scientists and clinicians. These courses would embrace the precepts of learner-centered teaching discussed earlier. This problem-oriented program would include attention to such topics as the doctor-patient relationship and physical exam and diagnostic skills. It would offer medical students an opportunity to *integrate* and *apply* their basic and behavioral science knowledge to real problems. As discussed in Chapter 6, this application to real-life problems should enhance motivation as well as impart important attitudes and skills.

Factual information would be replaced by curricular content which emphasizes application, creativity and learning. The new preclinical curriculum would advance the principles of learner-centered medical education and address the current shortcomings recognized by educators:

> The principal aim in improving the preclinical curriculum should be to do what other professional schools did many years ago: reduce the amount of factual information conveyed in the classroom and employ teaching methods that emphasize problem solving and the mastery of basic principles rather than memorization of detail. (Bok, 1984, p. 41)

The potential benefits of a structure for medical training such as the one proposed is evidenced in the documented success or a few six-year combined college-medical school programs. Twenty of the nation's thirty-three medical schools who offer combined baccalaureate-M.D. programs require (or allow) six or seven years of study rather than the traditional eight it would take to finish college and medical school (Norman & Calkins, 1992). In these curricula, students learn material in their fourth year of college which is traditionally taught in the first year of medical school.

The argument that students who do not spend eight years in training (four in college, four in medical school) will not perform as well as others who do has not been substantiated by evaluation research. In fact, there is evidence to the contrary. Callahan et al. (1992) compared the academic records of students in a combined program with those in a traditional program at one medical school and found that the latter actually performed better. Jacobs, Hinkley and Pennell (1988) also found that students in the six-year accelerated program performed better than the students in the traditional program at the University of Miami. As Olson (1992) states:

> Nothing but tradition mandates that all students wishing to study medicine should spend exactly four academic years in college and wait until their fourth year to learn whether they will be admitted to medical school. (p. 783)

Without some form of standardization and quality control, it is difficult to seriously consider adoption of the proposed structure. As Olson (1992) states: "To be sure, medical schools admit students from so many different colleges and universities that it would be virtually impossible to establish an integrated program with all of them" (p. 784). If, however, the integration was accomplished through clearly defined and regulated national requirements for premedical and preclinical medical training, and if medical school applicants were required to demonstrate proficiency through standardized testing in the defined areas, then it would be feasible. Combining efforts to offer an integrated program of premedical and preclinical training which emphasizes the development of a solid foundation of knowledge followed by application, creativity, and life-long learning would truly reform and revitalize medical education.

The proposed consolidation of college prerequisites and preclinical curricula would force medical educators to reconsider the basic science requirements for medical training and most certainly, in the end, reduce the amount of *less meaningful* information in the curriculum. In light of what we know about the current curricular overload of information and the long-term validity and retention of such information, re-appraisal and adoption of a new structure are reform efforts which are long overdue. Several medical educators agree that the time has come to consider reducing the amount of wasted time spent in medical school (Inui, 1992). Some even support the argument that the goals and objectives of medical school can be met in three rather than four years (Inui, 1992; Ebert & Ginzberg, 1988). As Bok (1984) states, the arguments for maintaining the plethora of information within the current curricular structure are "shopworn and unconvincing" (p. 41). Instead of fostering motivation and instilling a set of attitudes favorable to the inquiring mind of the physician-to-be, we have been turning potential applicants off, burning students out, and, in the best of circumstances, overloading them with useless and forgettable facts.

In the newly structured curriculum, students would be prepared to enter their required rotations much earlier. Just as it is logical to combine premedical with preclinical training, it might also be beneficial to combine the last year of clinical training in medical school with the first year of residency (internship).

The current state of most medical school curricula in the fourth year involves electives and sub-internships. These learning experiences often are repeated in much greater depth during their next three years of training. As Inui (1992) states, "These latter experiences seem unnecessary, given the extensive experiences to be acquired in these same settings during the internships and other postgraduate residency years" (p. 35). To increase efficiency in teaching and learning (to avoid duplication and wasting time) and to expedite the process of increasing learners' responsibility for patient care, it makes sense to move students on to their residency soon after they finish their required medical school rotations. Recognition that the fourth year of medical school could be more productively spent in a residency program is supported by the decision of some schools to drop it in favor of a three-year curriculum (Bok, 1984).

Within the proposed structure, the required clerkships will need to be refined to ensure a *foundation* for advanced learning in residency, just as the proposed premedical curriculum would serve as a foundation for the application of knowledge in the first year of medical school.

To implement a new curricular structure along these lines would demand a concerted effort of all governing boards including the AAMC, AMA and other organizations responsible for the development and implementation of policy regarding curriculum. Several barriers could be anticipated. Initially, medical schools may be apprehensive about producing graduates faster, thus decreasing the applicant pool. Colleges may fear a loss of control over their curricular offerings to those students going into medicine and could experience increased pressure and cost while implementing such a program. Finally, traditional medical organizations, by their very nature, are slow to support change and to disrupt the status quo.

The first step in undertaking such a task is to convince the appropriate groups of the need for such an undertaking. To assume and suggest that the current system is replete with overlap and waste, and that the length of training is keeping some of the best and brightest college students from entering the profession, would not be enough. If such change is to be successfully initiated and implemented, it will have to be supported by the public. Two aspects of the proposed change in structure would be in the public interest: decreased public financing of medical education and increased attention to the primary health care needs of our nation.

One reason for initiating the combined baccalaureate/M.D. programs in the early 1960s was to reduce the cost of medical education (Norman & Calkins, 1992). Very little of the actual cost of educating a medical student in a traditional four-year program is paid by the student. Only 4.2 percent of the total revenues of a medical school are generated by tuition (Jolin et al., 1992). The remaining costs are absorbed by: (1) affiliated health care institutions which in turn are reflected in higher health care costs (thus higher insurance premiums); or (2) the government (viz., taxes) through a variety of subsidies to medical training programs.

Medical schools are supported primarily from public funds. By the end of the 1980s, the federal government alone subsidized 58 percent of medical schools' operating budgets either through federal grants or through contributions to group practices by medicare and medicaid (Stemmler, 1989). In 1990–91 federal funding from grants and contracts alone totaled over $3 billion (Jolin et al., 1992).

State taxes are also busily at work supporting medical education. In 1990–91 state and local government appropriations totaled over $2 billion (Jolin et al., 1992). All medical schools received an average of $21 million, or nearly 13 percent of total revenues from state and local government appropriations in 1990–1991. Public medical schools received an average of nearly $35 million, or 24 percent of their funding from state governments in 1990–91 (Jolly et al., 1993).

Medical schools also received a substantial portion of funding from affiliated hospitals and clinics. In 1990–91 this amounted to 11 percent of their total revenues: over $2 billion (Jolin et al., 1992).

If we were to take the total amount of subsidized cost for all medical training in one year (i.e., $7 billion) and consider that we will save this amount every four years in the national production of physicians, then the economic benefit to the nation is quite clear.

Another way to view the cost benefit is from the perspective of the medical student. If the student can save an average of $28,000 for one year of tuition and living costs, it would substantially reduce his/her future indebtedness and facilitate the process of him/her becoming a wage-earning and spending citizen. This would have a tremendous impact on future earning requirements and perhaps on the specialty choice of students. For example Petersdorf (1991) states that: "Student indebtedness of $50,000, slightly less than the mean indebtedness of all medical students in 1989, requires a five-year post-M.D. income level of $79,000 for repayment to be "comfortable" for the student" (p. 63). Jolin et al. (1992) report that the average indebtedness of all medical school graduates by 1991 actually was over $50,000. In fact, a memo from Petersdorf, to the Council of Deans (Oct. 20, 1992), reports mean indebtedness at $55,859 (an increase of $5,475 over the previous year). He concludes: "From these data it seems unlikely that, faced with the magnitude of repayment schedules, individuals can opt for anything other than high-paying medical careers. The alternative is massive default" (p. 63).

Kassebaum and Szenas (1992) agree that although, in general, educational debt is relatively uninfluential in determining specialty choice (6.2% rated debt as a strong influence), significant indebtedness (> $75,000) does exert strong influence on specialty choice for 13 percent of graduates. As indebtedness rises, students will most likely continue to choose higher-paying subspecialties. Lower indebtedness which results from fewer years in medical school would likely remove some financial barriers to the selection of primary care specialties.

The proposed curricular structure also would increase the number of primary care physicians in practice in another way. Recent research suggests that the proportion of primary care physicians, relative to other specialists, is small and that the actual number in practice is insufficient to meet our nation's needs. In addition, the trend is toward the production of fewer rather than more primary care physicians. Data indicate that, in 1991, 19 percent fewer U.S. medical graduates entered primary care specialties than in 1986 (Colwill, 1992). The Task Force for the AAMC on the Generalist Physician (1992) reports:

> The number of generalist physicians entering practice in the United States has declined markedly over the last several years even though the need for the services provided by such physicians has increased steadily. These divergent trends have engendered concern among health care policy experts with the result that schools of medicine and teaching hospitals are being challenged to find ways to encourage more students and residents to choose generalist careers. (p. 1)

Under the proposed curriculum structure, where students will finish in three years rather than four years, even if the proportion of those going into primary care remains constant, the number of students going into primary care will increase in the short run. Using current figures, after three years we will have graduated an additional class of medical students, 20 percent of whom enter primary care specialties. This is a significant rationale for the proposed structural change.

The notion that a more streamlined curriculum could produce more primary care physicians to improve the health care delivery in this country is not new. In fact, it was a strong incentive to develop new combined baccalaureate/M.D. programs during the 1970s (Norman & Calkins, 1992). The time has come to reconsider adopting such a curricular structure on a national level.

One potential argument against the proposed curricular structure is that we would produce more physicians than are needed. However, we can be confident that inertia within our health care system, which is driven by the laws of supply and demand, would drive students to choose a specialty which not only is personally desirable but also offers the greatest opportunity for building a successful practice. In the foreseeable future the inertia would be in the direction of primary care.

If we perpetuate a curricular structure which is wasteful and crammed with irrelevant material for the sake of *keeping the applicant pool high* or *not overproducing physicians,* then medical education will not succeed in meeting its goals. Chances become greater that highly qualified college students may choose other professions because of the length and perceived repetitiveness of the curriculum. If we fail to create such structural reform of curriculum which is well thought out, planned for years in advance, and based on sound educational principle, change may be initiated by others outside of medicine and medical education with different motivations and goals.

Stemmler (1989), for example, presents one possible scenario where, because of financial considerations, the whole of basic science training breaks off from the medical school domain and becomes the responsibility of the colleges and universities. In such a situation, clinical faculty will be torn by a greater need to subsidize their salaries with clinical revenues and by the need to teach even more. At the same time, the federal government may become more involved in the medical education system to ensure the production of more primary care physicians.

GOALS OF THE CURRICULUM

Like other institutions of higher education, and indeed, all other organizations, medical schools are guided by aims and goals. Although there may be some variation in emphasis based on philosophy from one institution to the next, there is a great deal of commonality among medical schools in this area. The overriding aim of the medical school, like any other organization, is to survive in order to accomplish its goals. This means possessing the human and other resources necessary to carry out its strategies or functions.

In the broadest sense medical schools have three goals: teaching, research and patient care (not necessarily in that order). It is clear that these goals can often be in competition and conflict with each other (Bussigel et al., 1988). The conflict is often the result of trying to meet the basic aim of survival and, though not explicit, is created by forces outside of the institution. Once in motion these conflicts adversely affect the well-being of the institution. For example, currently there is a trend nationally to freeze or cut federal and state appropriations and grants to medical schools (Jolin, 1992a). Medical schools are forced to pass the cuts along to departments, which, depending on whether they are basic or clinical, are forced to look for new sources of revenues. Basic scientists are forced to write more grants. Clinical faculty are forced to see more patients. This inhibits teaching in the classroom, laboratory, or clinic and at the bedside, or at rounds.

The dramatic increases in operating revenues of medical schools from practice plans (from nearly sixteen to nearly thirty-two percent between 1981 and 1991) and hospital/clinics (from about six to nearly eleven percent) during the same period (Jolin, 1992) reflect this trend toward clinical activity and a commensurate shift in the relative importance placed on each of these three goals.

Medical schools are conflicted because of their inability to precisely define and meet each of these three goals. The importance of teaching is self-evident. However, this is the most expensive of the three goals. It is labor intensive and there is very little financial return. Research and patient care, on the other hand, both can generate substantial financial reward and prestige for the institution. Their role in helping the institution to achieve its basic aim to survive makes *them* more important. Faculty are encouraged (covertly as well as overtly) to meet these goals, and those that succeed possess leverage with respect to their profession (salary, promotion, tenure, etc.).

It is clear that if medical education is to survive, then recognition and resolution of this conflict of goals is necessary. It must be accomplished at all levels in the system with increased support for teaching. Adequate federal and state appropriations should be designated for medical teaching and sustained with the realization that the medical school cannot make up shortfalls using patient care or research funds without severely detracting from the teaching mission.

Funding from state and federal sources should be distributed equitably among each of the one hundred and thirty-three medical schools. It can be calculated as the difference between revenue necessary to support teaching and the money available to the institution for teaching from tuition, training grants, endowment income, etc. This financial support would be considered *teaching money* by the institution *and* by the state or federal government. Changes in the amount of support should be made with the realization that they will directly affect the teaching program.

The first step in implementing these changes will be to educate state and federal representatives about the necessity of maintaining separateness among the three goals. In a reciprocal fashion, institutions will have to commit to the amount of teaching time which they have defined. Monitoring implementation of such a program will demand the assistance of organizations like the AAMC.

Medical schools will have to make other structural changes to achieve the goal of excellence in teaching. There should be provisions for faculty with advanced skills, experience and interest in teaching, to engage more fully in the achievement of this goal. As mentioned earlier, these faculty should be recognized on a par with faculty whose strengths are research or patient care. Specifically, salary and appointment levels of faculty involved in teaching and those involved in research should be comparable.

Other aspects of recognition, such as tenure and promotion, should be equally attainable by faculty choosing different paths. As previously mentioned, it is no secret that research has traditionally been the determining factor in these decisions and that teaching holds little weight. The *age-old* argument that there are not enough objective criteria to document excellence in teaching is unsubstantiated. All medical journals publish articles on teaching; some are devoted totally to this topic. In addition, many training grants offer the opportunity to develop innovative teaching programs, and countless opportunities exist to present innovative educational projects at national meetings. Promotion and tenure committees must be creative in determining the specific criteria for such a system of formal recognition. These criteria must be rigorous and meaningful.

SUMMARY OF PART III

There is substantial evidence that medical education is not healthy (viz., functioning optimally). The current emphasis on curricular reform nationally must be accompanied by a broader perspective which includes the medical school environment. This entails the development of a learner and teacher-centered climate, an appropriate curricular structure, and a balanced orientation toward teaching, research and patient care. Only when these aspects of the environment are addressed will we be able to effect true learner-centered medical education.

BIBLIOGRAPHY

AAMC Report, *Medical School Admissions Requirements,* 1993–94, United States and Canada (43rd ed). Washington, D.C., Assoc Am Med Colleges, 1992.

AAMC Report, *Medical School Admissions Requirements,* 1991–92, United States and Canada (41st ed). Washington, D.C., Assoc Am Med Colleges, 1990.

AAMC Special Advisory Panel on Technical Standards for Medical School Admission; Letter approved for transmittal by AAMC Executive Council, January 18, 1978.

Aaron, P.G., and Phillips, S.: A decade of research with dyslexic college students: A summary of findings. *Ann Dyslexia, 36:*44–66, 1986.

Accardo, P., Haake, C., Whitman, B.: The learning-disabled medical student. *J Devel Beh Pedi, 10:*253–258, 1989.

Adams, J.A.: *Human Memory.* New York, McGraw-Hill, 1967.

Adsett, A.: Psychological health of medical students in relation to the medical education process. *J Med Educ, 43:*728–734, 1968.

Alpert, R., and Haber, R.N.: Anxiety in academic achievement situations. *J Abn Soc Psych, 61:*207–215, 1960.

American Psychiatric Assn., DSM–III, 1980.

Annis, L.F.: Effect of cognitive style and learning passage organization on study technique effectiveness. *J Educ Psychol, 71:*620–6, 1979.

Annis, L.F., and Davis, K.J.: Study technique and cognitive style: Their effect on recall and recognition. *J Educ Rsrch, 71:*175–178, 1977.

Ashikawa, H., Hojat, M., Zeleznik, C., and Gonnella, J.S.: Reexamination of relationships between students' undergraduate majors, medical school performances, and career plans at Jefferson Medical College. *Acad Med, 66:*458–464, 1991.

Barrows, H.S.: Comments: The clinical teacher and the learning process. In Gastel, B., and Rogers, D.E.: *Clinical Education and the Doctor of Tomorrow.* New York, NY Acad of Medicine, 1989, pp. 47–52.

Barrows, Howard S.: *How to Design a Problem-based Curriculum for the Preclinical Years.* New York, Springer, 1985.

Bartlett, F.: *Thinking.* London, George Allen & Unwin Ltd., 1958.

Bartlett, F.: *Remembering.* London, Cambridge U Press, 1961.

Bellezza, F.S.: Mnemonic devices: Classification, characteristics, and criteria. *Rev Educ Rsrch, 51:*247–275, 1981.

Berger, E., and Goldberger, L.: Field dependence and short-term memory. *Perceptual and Motor Skills, 49:*87–96, 1979.

Bertini, M.: Some implications of field dependence for education. In Bertini, M., Pizzamigleo, L., and Wapner, S. (eds): *Field Dependence in Psychological Theory,*

Research, and Application. Hillsdale NJ, Lawrence Erlbaum Assoc, 1986, pp. 93–106.

Bhushan, V., Chu, E., and Hansen, J.: *First Aid for the Boards.* Norwalk CT, Appleton & Lange, 1993.

Billings, J.S.: Methods of research in medical literature. *Trans Assoc Am Physicians,* 2:57–67, 1887.

Bishop, C.W.: Teaching diagnosis by computer. *Physiologist, 28:*451, 1985.

Blois, Marsden S.: *Information and Medicine.* Berkeley, U.CA Press, 1984.

Bloom, B.S., Hastings, J.T., and Madqus, G.F.: *Handbook on Formative and Summative Evaluation of Student Learning.* New York, McGraw-Hill, 1971.

Bloom, S.W.: Medical education in transition: Paradigm change and organizational stasis. In Marston, R.Q., and Jones, R.M.: *Medical Education in Transition.* Princeton NJ, Robert Wood Johnson Foundation, 1992, pp. 15–25.

Bok, Derek: A new way to train doctors. *Harvard Magazine,* May–June, pp. 32–71, 1984.

Boshuizen, H.P.A., and Schmidt, H.G.: The developing structure of medical knowledge. In Nooman, Z.M., Schmidt, H.G., and Ezzat, E.S., (eds): *Innovation in Medical Education: An Evaluation of Its Present Status.* New York, Springer, 1990, pp. 218–240.

Brinkman, E.H.: Programmed instruction and a technique for improving spatial visualization. *J Applied Psych, 50:*179–184, 1966.

Brooks, L.W., Dansereau, D.F., Spurlin, J.E., and Holley, C.D.: Effects of headings on text processing. *J Educ Psych, 75:*292–302, 1983.

Brooks, J.B., and Stoney, S.D.: Motor mechanisms: The role of the pyramidal system in motor control. *Ann Rev Physiol, 33:*337–392, 1971.

Bruner, J.S.: *Toward a Theory of Instruction.* Cambridge MA, Belknap Press, 1971.

Bruner, J.S.: *On Knowing Essays for the Left Hand.* Cambridge MA, Belknap Press, 1962.

Bruner, J.S.: The act of discovery. *Harv Educ Rev, 31:*21–32, 1961.

Bruner, J.S.: *The Process of Education.* New York, Vintage Books, pp. 25–32, 1960.

Bureau of Study Counsel: *Managing Your Time: Hints On How To Beat Procrastination.* Cambridge MA, Harv U, 1984.

Bussigel, M.N., Barzansky, B.M., and Grenholm, G.G.: *Innovation Processes in Medical Education.* New York, Praeger, 1988.

Byrne, P., and Long, B.: *Doctors Talking to Patients.* London, HMSO, 1978.

Callahan, C., Vleoski, J.J., Xu G., Hojat, M., Zeleznik, Gonella, J.K.: The Jefferson-Penn State B.S.-M.D. program: a 26 year experience. *Acad Med, 76:*792–7, 1992.

Canady, S.D., and Lancaster, C.J.: Impact of undergraduate courses on medical students performance in basic sciences. *J Med Educ, 60:*757–763, 1985.

Cantor, J.C., et al.: Medical educators' views on medical education reform. *JAMA, 265:*1002–6, 1991.

Cermack, L.S.: *Improving Your Memory.* New York, McGraw-Hill, 1975.

Cochran, K.F., and Davis, K.J.: Individual differences in inference processes. *J of Research in Personality, 21:*197–210, 1987.

Collins, A., and Brown, J.S.P.: The computer as a tool for learning through reflection.

In *Learning Issues for Intelligent Tutoring Systems.* New York, Springer-Verlag, 1988.

Collen, M.F.: *Hospital Computer Systems.* New York, J Wiley and Sons, 1974.

Colwill, J.M.: Where have all the primary care applicants gone? *N Engl J Med, 326:*387–393, 1992.

Crutchfield, R.S.: Nurturing the cognitive skills of productive thinking. In Rubin, L.J. (ed): *Life Skills in School and Society.* Assoc Superv & Curric Dev 1969 Yearbook, Washington DC, 1969, pp. 53–72.

Davis, J.K.: Educational implications of field dependence-independence. In Wapner, S., and Demick, J. (eds): *Field Dependence-Independence.* Hillsdale NJ, Lawrence Erlbaum Assoc, 1991, pp. 149–176.

Davis, J.K., and Cochran, K.F.: An information processing view of field dependence-independence. *Early Childhood Development and Care, 51:*31–47, 1989.

Davis, J.K.: The field independent-dependent cognitive style and beginning reading. *Early Childhood Development and Care, 29:*119–132, 1987.

Davis, J.K., and Frank, B.M.: Learning and memory of field independent-dependent individuals. *J Rsrch Personality, 13:*469–479, 1979.

Davis, Neil: *Medical Abbreviations,* 8600, 6th ed, Canada, NM Davis Assoc, 1990.

Dean, J.M.: Heartlab, *MD Computing, 4:*46–49, 1987.

Dixon, Roger A., and Hertzog, C.: A functional approach to memory and metamemory development in adulthood. In Weinert, F.E., and Perlmutter, M. (eds): *Memory Development: Universal Changes and Individual Differences.* Hillsdale NJ, Lawrence Erlbaum Assoc, 1988, pp. 293–330.

Doblin, B., and Korenman, S.: The role of natural science in the premedical curriculum. *Acad Med, 67:*539–541, 1992.

Ebert, R.H., and Ginzberg, E.: The reform of medical education. *Health Affairs, 7:*5–9, 1988.

Eisenberg, L.: Science in medicine: Too little and too limited in scope. *Am J Med, 84:*485, March, 1988.

Ellis, A.W.: The cognitive neuropsychology of developmental (and acquired) dyslexia: a critical survey. *Cognitive Neuropsychology, 2:*169–205, 1985.

Elstein, A.S., Kagan, N., Shulman, L.S., Jason, H., and Loupe, M.J.: Methods and theory in the study of medical inquiry. *J Med Educ, 47:*85–92, 1972.

Faigel, H.C.: Services for students with learning disabilities in U.S. and Canadian medical schools. *Acad Med, 67:*338–9, 1992.

Finger, R., and Galassi, J.P.: Effects of modifying cognitive versus emotionality responses in the treatment of test anxiety. *J Consulting Clin Psych, 45:*280–7, 1977.

Fisher, L.A., and Cotsonas Jr., N.J.: A time study of student activities. *J Med Educ, 40:*125–131, 1965.

Flavell, J.H.: *Cognitive Development.* Englewood Cliffs, Prentice-Hall, 1977.

Flexner, Abraham: *Medical Education, A Comparative Study.* New York, MacMillan Co, 1925.

Frank, B.M.: Effect of field independence-dependence and study technique on learning from a lecture. *J Am Educ Research, 21:*669–678, 1984.

Frank, B.M.: Flexibility of information processing and the memory of field-independent and field-dependent learners. *J Research in Personality, 17:*89–96, 1983.

Friedman, C.F., Twarag, R.R., Youngblood, P.L. and deBliek, R.: Computer databases as an educational tool in the basic sciences. *Acad Med,* 65:15–16, 1990.

Frierson Jr., H.T., and Hoban, D.: Effects of test anxiety on performance on the NBME Part I Examination. *J Med Educ, 62:*431–3, 1987.

Gardner, H.: *Frames of Mind.* New York, Basic Books, 1983.

Garfinkel, P.E., and Waring, E.M.: Personality, interests, and emotional disturbance in psychiatric residents. *Am J Psychiatry, 138:*51–5, 1981.

Garrard, J., Lorents, A., and Chilgren, R.: Student allocation of time in a semioptional medical curriculum. *J Med Educ, 47:*460–6, 1972.

Gibson, E.J.: *Principles of Perceptual Learning and Perceptual Behavior.* New York, New Appleton-Century Croft, 1969.

Goodenough, D.R.: History of the field dependence construct. In Bertini, M., Pizzamiglio, L., and Wapner, S. (eds), *Field Dependence in Psychological Theory, Research, and Application.* Hillsdale NJ, Lawrence Erlbaum Assoc, 1986, pp. 5–14.

Goodenough, D.R., Oltman, P.K., Freidman, F., Moore, C.A., Witkin, H.A., Owen, D., and Raskin, E.: Cognitive styles in the development of medical careers. *J Voc Beh, 14:*341–351, 1979.

Gregg, Alan: *For Future Doctors.* Chicago IL, U Chicago Press, 1957.

Gross, R.: *Peak Learning.* Los Angeles, J.P. Tarcher, 1991.

Guilford, J.P.: Factors that aid and hinder creativity. *Teachers Coll Rec, 63:*380–392, 1962.

Guyer, B.P.: Dyslexic doctors. *N Engl J Med, 321:*171, 1987.

Guyer, B.P.: Dyslexic doctors: A resource in need of discovery. *South Med J, 81:*1151–4, 1988.

Harris, A.J., and Sippay, E.R.: *How to Increase Reading Ability.* New York, Longman, 1990.

Holding, D.H.: Skills research. In Holding, D.H. (ed): *Human Skills.* New York, J Wiley & Sons, 1981, pp. 1–14.

Howell, C.C., and Swanson, S.C.: The relative influence of identified components of test anxiety in baccalaureate nursing students. *J Nsg Educ, 28:*215–220, 1989.

Hsu, K., and Marshall, V.: Prevalence of depression and distress in a large sample of Canadian residents, interns and fellows. *Am J Psychol, 144:*1561–5, 1987.

Inui, T., Carter, W., Kukul, W., and Haigh, V.: Outcome-based doctor-patient interaction analysis. *Med Care, 20:*6, 1982.

Inui, T.S.: The social contract and the medical school's responsibilities. In White, K.L., and Connelly, J.E. (eds), *The Medical School's Mission and the Population's Health.* New York, Springer-Verlag, 1992.

Jacobs, J.P., Hinkley, R.E., and Pennell, J.P.: Student evaluation of accelerated program at the University of Miami. *J Med Educ, 63:*11–18, 1988.

Jessee, W.F., and Simon, H.J.: Time utilization by medical students on a pass/fail evaluation system. *J Med Educ, 46:*275–280, 1971.

Johnson III, J.E., and Shuster, A.L.: Preparing physicians for the future. In Marston, R.Q., and Jones, R.M. (eds): *Medical Education in Transition.* Princeton NJ, The Robert Wood Johnson Foundation, 1992, pp. 26–41.

Johnson-Laird, P.N., and Wason, P.C.: *Thinking.* Cambridge, Cambridge U Press, 1980.

Jolin, L.D., Jolly, P., Krakower, J.Y., and Beran, R.S.: US medical school finances. *JAMA, 268:*1149–1155, 1992.

Jolly, P., Jolin, L.D., Beran, R.L., and Sanderson, S.C.: Medical school financing: comparing different types of schools and departments. *Acad Med, 68:*92–101, 1993.

Jones, E.E.: *Interpersonal Perception.* New York, WH Freeman and Co, 1990.

Just, M.A., and Carpenter, P.A.: Eye fixation and cognitive processes. *Cognitive Psych, 8:*441–480, 1976.

Kassebaum, D.G., and Szenas, P.L.: Relationship between indebtedness and specialty choices of graduating medical students. *Acad Med, 67:*700–7, 1992.

Kassirer, J.P., and Gorry, G.A.: Clinical problem solving: a behavioral analysis. *Ann Intern Med, 89:*245–255, 1978.

Knowles, Malcolm: *The Modern Practice of Adult Education.* Cambridge, Adult Educ Co NY, 1980.

Knowles, Malcolm: *Self-directed Learning: a Guide for Learners and Teachers.* Chicago, Follet, 1975.

Kolb, D.A.: Learning styles and disciplinary differences. In Chickering, A.W., and Assoc. (eds): *The Modern American College.* San Francisco, Jossey-Bass Pub, 1981, pp. 232–255.

Kolb, D.A.: *The Learning Style Inventory: Technical Manual.* Boston, McBer, 1976.

Liubomir, E., Radovanic, Z., Jevremovic, I., Marinkovic, J.: Psychiatric disorders and selected variables among medical students in Belgrade (Yugoslavia). *Soc Sci Med, 27:*187–190, 1988.

Luria, A.R.: *The Mind of a Mnemonist.* Cambridge MA, Harvard U Press, 1987.

Lyon, H.C., Healy, J.C., Bell, J.R., O'Donnell, J.F., Shultz, E.K., Wigton, R.S., Hirai, F., and Beck, J.R.: Significant efficiency findings while controlling for the frequent confounders of CAI research in the PlanAlyzer project's computer-based, self-paced, case-based programs in anemia and chest pain diagnosis. *J Med Systems, 15:*117–131, 1991.

Macan, T.H., Shahani, C., Dipboye, R.L., and Phillips, A.P.: College students' time management; correlations with academic performance and stress. *J Educ Psych, 82:*760–8, 1990.

Mandel, H.G.: The R.W. Johnson report: misguided reform of the basic sciences curriculum [letter]. *Acad Med, 68:*202, 1993.

Mandler, G., and Sarason, S.B.: A study of anxiety and learning. *J Abn Psych, 47:*166–173, 1954.

Mangione, S., Nieman, L.Z., Greenspon, L.W., and Margulies, H.: A comparison of computer-assisted instruction and small-group teaching of cardiac auscultation to medical students. *Med Educ, 25*(5):389–395, 1991.

Marteniuk, R.G.: The role of eye and head positions in slow movement execution. In Stelmach, G.E. (ed): *Information Processing in Motor Control and Learning.* New York, Academic Press, 1978, pp. 267–288.

Maslow, A.: *Toward a Psychology of Being.* New York, D Van Nostrand Co, 1968.

McAuliffe, W.E., Rohman, M., Santangelo, S., Feldman, B., Magnuson, E., Sobol, A., and Weissman, J.: Psychoactive drug use among practicing physicians and medical students. *N Engl J Med, 315:*805–810, 1986.

McMurray, J., Fitzgerald, E., and Bean, S.: Stress and support systems in preclinical medical students. *J Med Educ, 55:*216, 1980.

Mellinkoff, S.M.: Chemical intervention. *Scientific American, 229:*102–12, 1973.

Messick, S., and Witkin, H.: The meaning of style. In Bertini, M., Pizzamiglio, L., and Wapner, S. (eds): *Field Dependence in Psychological Theory, Research and Application.* Hillsdale NJ, Lawrence Erlbaum Assoc, 1986, pp. 115–118.

Miller, W.S.: *Word Wealth.* New York, Holt, Rinehart and Winston, 1967.

Miller, G.A. (ed): *Teaching and Learning in Medical School.* Cambridge MA, Harvard U Press, 1961.

Miller, G.A.: The magical number seven, plus or minus two: some limits on our capacity for processing information. *Psych Rev, 63:*81–97, 1956.

Moore, H.A., Goodenough, D.R., and Cox, P.W.: Field dependent and field independent cognitive styles and their educational implications. *Rev Educ Research, 47:*1–64, 1977.

Nardone, D.A., Schriner, C.L., Guyer-Kelley, P., and Kositch, L.P.: Use of computer simulations to teach history-taking to first year medical students. *J Med Educ, 62:*191–3, 1987.

Naus, M.J., Ornstein, P.A.: Development of memory strategies: Analysis questions and issues. In Chi, Michelene T.H. (ed), *Trends in Memory Development Research.* Basel; New York; Karger Pub, 1983.

Netter, F.H.: *Atlas of Human Anatomy.* West Cladwell NJ, CBA–GEIGY Co, 1989.

Neufield, V.R., Bearpark, S., and Winterton, C.: Optimal outcomes of clinical education. In Gastel, B., and Rogers, D.E. (eds): *Clinical Education and the Doctor of Tomorrow.* New York, New York Acad of Medicine, 1989, pp. 11–23.

Newell, K.M.: Skill learning. In Holding, D.H. (ed): *Human Skills.* New York, John Wiley and Sons, 1981, pp. 203–226.

Newell, K.M., and Shapiro, D.C.: Variability of practice and transfer of training; some evidence towards a schema view of motor learning. *J Motor Beh, 8:*233–243, 1976.

Nickerson, R.S.: Reasoning. In Dillon, R.F., and Sternberg, R.J. (eds): *Cognition and Instruction.* Orlando, Academic Press, 1986, pp. 343–374.

Nickerson, R.S., Perkins, D.N., and Smith, E.E.: *The Teaching of Thinking.* Hillsdale NJ, Lawrence Erlbaum Assoc, 1985.

Norman, A.W., and Calkins, E.V.: Curricular variations in combined baccalaureate/MD programs. *Acad Med, 67:*785–791, 1992.

Olson, D.R., and Bialystok, E.: *Spatial Cognition.* Hillsdale NJ, Lawrence Erlbaum Assoc, 1983.

Olson, S.W.: Combined-degree programs: a valuable alternative for motivated students who choose medicine early. *Acad Med, 67:*783–4, 1992.

Ornstein, P., Baker-Ward, A., and Naus, M.: The development of mnemonic skill. In Weinert, F.E., and Perlmutter, M. (eds): *Memory Development: Universal Changes and Individual Differences.* Hillsdale NJ, Lawrence Erlbaum Assoc, 1988.

Palmer, S.E.: Hierarchical structure in perceptual representation. *Cognitive Psych,* 9:441–474, 1977.

Petersdorf, R.G.: Memo from the president of the AAMC to the council of deans. October 20, 1992.

Petersdorf, R.G.: Financing medical education. *Acad Med, 66:*65–6, 1991.

Phifferling, J., Blum, J., and Wood, W.: Physician impairment. *J Kansas Med Soc, 82:*509–515, 1981.

Quirk, M.E., Ciottone, R., Letendre, D., and Wapner, S.: Critical person-in-environment transitions in medical education. *Med Teacher, 9:*415–423, 1987.

Quirk, M.E., and Letendre, A.: Teaching communication skills to first year medical students. *J Med Educ, 61:*603–5, 1986.

Quirk, M.E., and Babineau, R.A.: Teaching interviewing skills to students in clinical years: a comparative analysis of three strategies. *J Med Educ, 57:*939–941, 1982.

Rappleye, W.: *Medical Education: The Final Report of the Commission on Medical Education.* New York, Association of American Medical Colleges, 1932.

Raskin, E.: Counseling implications of field dependence-independence in an educational setting. In Bertini, M., Pizzamiglio, L., and Wapner, S. (eds): *Field Dependence in Psychological Theory, Research and Application.* Hillsdale NJ, L Erlbaum Assoc, 1986, pp. 107–114.

Reardon, R., Jolly, E.J., McKinney, K.D., and Forducy, P.: Field dependence/independence and active learning of verbal and geometric material. *Perceptual Motor Skills, 55:*263–6, 1982.

Richardson, A.: Mental practice: A review and discussion. *Rsch Quarterly, 38:*95–107, 1967.

Rochford, K.: Spatial learning disabilities and underachievement among university anatomy students. *Med Educ, 19:*13–26, 1985.

Rogers, C.: *Humanizing Education: the Person in the Process.* Washington DC, Assn for Superv and Curric Devel, 1967.

Rogers, C.R.: *Freedom to Learn.* Columbus, CE Merrill, 1969.

Russell, A.T., Pasnau, R.O., and Taintor, Z.C.: Emotional problems of residents in psychiatry. *Am J Psychiatry, 132:*263–7, 1975.

Sarason, S.B., Mandler, G., and Craighill, P.G.: The effect of differential instructions on anxiety and learning. *J Abn Psych, 47:*561–565, 1952.

Schroeder, S.A., Zones, J.S., and Showstack, J.A.: Academic medicine as a public trust. *JAMA, 262:*803–812, 1989.

Scriven, M.: The methodology of evaluation. *AERA Monograph Series on Curriculum Evaluation, #1:*39–83, 1967.

Shain, D.D.: *Study Skills and Test-taking Strategies for Medical Students: Oklahoma Notes.* New York, Springer-Verlag, 1992.

Simek-Downing, L., and Quirk, M.: Videotape analyses of medical students' interviewing skills. *Fam Med, 17:*57–60, 1985.

Simpson, M.A.: *Medical Education: A Critical Approach.* London, Butterworths, 1972.

Smith, L.H.: Medical education for the 21st century. *J Med Educ,* 60:106–112, 1985.

Smith, R.C.: Teaching interviewing skills to medical students: The issue of 'counter-transference'. *J Med Educ, 59:*582–7, 1984.

Snodgrass, J.G., and Hirshman, E.: Dissociations among implicit and explicit memory tasks: the role of stimulus similarity. *J Exp Psych: Learning, Memory and Cognition, 2:*150–160, 1994.

Spielberger, C.D., Anton, W., and Bedell, J.R.: The nature and treatment of test anxiety. In Spielberger, C.D., and Zuckerman, M. (eds): *Emotions and Anxiety; New Concepts, Methods and Applications.* New York, Lawrence Erlbaum/Wiley, 1976.

Spiro, R.J., and Tirre, W.C.: Individual differences in schema utilization during discourse processing. *J Educ Psych, 72:*204–8, 1980.

Spurlin, J., Collins-Eiland, K., and Dansereau, D.: *Cognitive learning strategies series for medical students.* Volume III: Strategies for Taking Tests and Reducing Test Anxiety. Spurlin, Galveston, Collins-Eiland and Dansereau Pub, 1984.

Stemmler, E.J.: The Medical School—Where does it go from here? *Acad Med, 64:*182–5, 1989.

Sternberg, R.G.: *Intelligence in the Psychology of Human Thought.* Cambridge, Cambridge U Press, 1988.

Stillman, P.L., Regan, M.B., Swanson, D.B., Case, S., McCahan, J., Feinblatt, J., Smith, S.R., Willms, J., and Nelson, D.V.: An assessment of the clinical skills of fourth-year students at four New England medical schools. *Acad Med, 65:*320–6, 1990.

Stillman, P.L., Madigan, H.S., Thompson, D.K., Swanson, D.B., Julian, E., Regan, M.B., Nelson, V., and Philbin, M.: The Medical Education Evaluation Program of the state of Ohio. *Acad Med, 64:*454–7, 1989.

Stokols, D.: Environment psychology. *Ann Rev Psychol, 29:*253–295, 1978.

Stone, H.L., Meyer, T.C., and Shilling, R.: Alternative medical school curriculum design: An independent study program. *Med Teacher, 13:*149–156, 1991.

Stryer, L.: *Biochemistry.* New York, WH Freeman & Co, 1988.

Suchman, Richard J.: The child and the inquiry process. In Passaw, A.H., and Leeper, R.R. (eds): *Intellectual Development: Another Look,* Washington D.C., ASCD, 1964, pp. 59–77.

Swanson, A.G., and Anderson, M.B.: Educating medical students: ACME–TRI Report. *Acad Med, 68:*S7–S48, 1993.

Taylor, C.R.: Great expectations: the reading habits of year II medical students. *N Engl J Med, 326:*1436–40, 1992.

Thomas, C.B.: What becomes of medical students: the dark side. *J Jhn Hop Med, 138:*185–196, 1976.

Thomas, L.: *The Youngest Science: Notes of a Medicine-Watcher.* New York, Viking, 1983.

Thomas, L.: Notes of a biology-watcher. How to fix the premedical curriculum. *N Engl J Med, 298:*1180–1, 1978.

Thompson, L.J.: Part III: the dyslexic child grows up: language disabilities in men of eminence. *Bull Orton Soc,* pp. 113–120, 1969.

Tooth, D., Tonge, K., and McManus, I.C.: Anxiety and study methods in preclinical students: Causal relation to examination performance. *Med Educ, 23:*416–21, 1989.

Tulving, E.: *Elements of Episodic Memory.* New York, Oxford U Press, 1983.

Tyler, Ralph: *Basic Principles of Curriculum and Instruction.* Chicago IL, Chicago U Press, 1950.

Valko, R.J., and Clayton, P.J.: Depression in the internship. *Dis Nerv Syst, 36:*26–9, 1975.

Verbeek, H.A.: Self-instruction through patient simulation by computer. *Med Educ, 21:*10–14, 1987.

Vinacke, W.E.: *The Psychology of Thinking.* New York, McGraw-Hill, 1952.

Wapner, Seymour, and Demick, J. (eds): *Some Open Research Problems on Field Dependence-Independence in Field Dependence-Independence.* Hillsdale NJ, Lawrence Erlbaum Assoc, 1991.

Wapner, S.: A holistic, developmental, systems-oriented environmental psychology: some beginnings. In Stokols, D., and Altman, I. (eds): *Handbook of Environmental Psychology.* New York, John Wiley, 1987.

Waring, E.M.: Emotional illness in psychiatric trainees. *Br J Psychiatry, 125:*10–11, 1974.

Webster, Noah: *Webster's New Collegiate Dictionary.* Springfield MA, G&G Merriam Co, 1977.

Whitehead, Alfred North: *The Aims of Education and Other Essays.* New York, The Free Press, 1929.

Willey, M.S., and Jarecky, B.M.: *Analysis and Application of Information.* U Maryland School of Med, 1976.

Williams, I.D., and Rodney, M.: Intrinsic feedback, interpolation, and the closed-loop theory. *J Motor Beh, 10:*25–36, 1978.

Witkin, H.A., and Goodenough, D.R.: *Cognitive Styles: Essence and Origins. Field Dependence and Independence.* New York, International Universities Press, 1981.

Witkin, H.A., Moore, C.A., Oltman, P.K., Goodenough, D.R., Friedman, F., Owen, D.R., and Raskin, E.: The role of the field dependent and field independent cognitive styles in academic evolution: A longitudinal study. *J Educ Psych, 69:*197–211, 1977.

Witkin, H.A., Oltman, P.K., Raskin, E., and Karp, S.A.: *Manual for Embedded Figures Test, Children's Embedded Figures Test and Group Embedded Figures Test.* Palo Alto CA, Consulting Psychologists Press, 1971.

Wolf, F.M., Ulman, J.G., Saltzman, G.A., and Savickas, M.L.: Allocation of time and perceived coping behavior of first-year medical students. *J Med Educ, 55:*956–8, 1980.

Wolf, T.M., Von Almen, T.K., Faucett, J.M., Randall, H.M., and Franklin, F.A.: Psychosocial changes during the first year of medical school. *Med Educ, 25:*174–181, 1991.

Yates, F.A.: *The Art of Memory.* London, Routledge & Kegan Paul, 1966.

AUTHOR INDEX

SUBJECT INDEX

201